50¢

Your
Body,
Yourself

Your Body, Yourself

a guide to your changing body

by Alison Bell and Lisa Rooney, M.D.
reviewed and updated by Doreen Virtue, Ph.D.

LOWELL HOUSE JUVENILE

LOS ANGELES

CONTEMPORY BOOKS
CHICAGO

To Jim, with love
—A.B.

To my family—for everything
—L.R.

Cataloging-in-Publication number is available.

Publisher: Jack Artenstein

Vice President and Associate Publisher: Elizabeth Amos
Director of Publishing Services: Rena Copperman
Editor-in-Chief, Nonfiction: Amy Downing
Cover Design: Lisa Theresa Lenthall
Text Design: Brenda Leach
Cover photograph: Ann Bogart
Model: Jenny Powers

ISBN: 1-56565-532-X

10   9   8   7   6   5   4   3   2

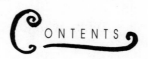

Contents

Your Body, Yourself is a book that will clear up a lot of questions you may have about growing up. However, no book can answer every question that might come up as you enter your teen years. If you have a question you need answered, don't be afraid to talk to an adult about it—especially your mom or dad! You may even want to sit down with a parent and read through parts of the book together.

This book is not intended to treat, diagnose, or prescribe. If you or anyone else has a serious health problem, we suggest that you consult a professional health worker.

Am I Normal to Be Feeling This Way?

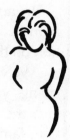

"I think what is happening to me is so wonderful, and not only what can be seen on my body, but all that is taking place inside."

—Anne Frank, *The Diary of a Young Girl*

You've probably heard that once you're into your teen years, life gets pretty crazy and confusing.

Then why, if you're not a teen yet (or just barely a teen), are you so confused sometimes? One minute you're up, the next you're down. One minute you think you're pretty great, the next you wonder why anybody would want to be your friend. One minute you can't wait to grow up, the next you wish you could stay a kid forever.

What's going on?

Something completely normal. Something that happens to every girl. You're growing up. You're not a teen yet, but you're not a kid either. You're an in-betweener. And that's a hard place to be!

7

Not only are your emotions yo-yoing, your body's changing, too. These physical and emotional changes are overwhelming. They can even be scary. That's what this book is for—to reassure you that you're okay and to answer all of your questions.

In this book, we tell you everything you ever wanted to know about growing up. We'll fill you in on all the changes you can expect your body to go through (on the outside and inside)—from your developing breasts to getting your period. We also set you straight about sex.

In addition, we've included chapters on nutrition, common health problems to be aware of, and the latest information on the three big baddies: drugs, alcohol, and smoking.

We've also devoted a chapter to all of those emotional swings you may be experiencing. We give tips on how to survive these crazy years without driving yourself, your friends, your family, and even your pet dog bonkers!

And in this updated edition, we've added more information on what *you* want to know about—eating disorders, exercising, and even what you can expect at your first visit to the gynecologist.

We're also here to tell you that you're not alone. Every girl, including your mom, grandmother, school principal, and doctor, goes through this development process. The more you grow up, the more comfortable you'll feel about yourself. And remember this: There's so much to look forward to! Dances, school football games, meeting new friends, dating, getting your driver's license. It's all in your future. And it's all a lot of fun.

So, take heart. You're about to enter the best years of your life.

Alison Bell   Lisa B. Rooney

$\mathcal{W}$hy Am I Changing?

"She could never be really sure of anything this summer. One moment she was happy, and the next, for no reason, she was miserable. An hour ago she had loved her sneakers, now she detested them."

—Sara Godfrey in Betsy Byars's The Summer of the Swans

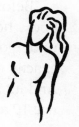

$\mathcal{A}$lmost overnight, you begin changing so fast your head may spin! For starters, your body's changing. Your breasts are developing, which can make you feel self-conscious. You discover hair in places you never thought you'd see it. And horrors—you might have even discovered your first pimple!

You're also wrestling with new and powerful feelings. Those boys who used to be pests or pals may now start looking pretty cute. You might even be in the middle of your first crush. Your feelings toward old girlfriends may be on a roller-coaster ride, too. You may find you'd rather meet new friends than hang out with your old ones. At home, you want to be alone more. You love your family but need your privacy.

What's going on? It's all part of a process called *puberty*.

What Is Puberty?

Puberty is a signal that your body is maturing. While you may not plan on having children for 10 or even 20 years, your body is getting ready to produce babies. Puberty usually begins between the ages of 8 and 14. (The average age is 10½.)

How does it all start? Puberty has a lot to do with the chemical substances in your body called *hormones*.

Before you even notice any outward changes in your body, hormones are at work inside your body. Your body undergoes many internal transformations. No one knows exactly what triggers or sets the hormones of puberty flowing. And it's still a mystery as to why puberty begins in one girl at age 10 and in another at age 13. But the sequence of events is the same. First, the part of your brain called the *hypothalamus* starts producing a special hormone called gonadotropin releasing hormone (GnRH). This hormone travels to another part of your brain called the *pituitary gland*. The pituitary gland then releases two other hormones, luteinizing hormone (LH) and follicle stimulating hormone (FSH) into your bloodstream, where they travel to your ovaries. From there, a whole chain of hormone production is now set in motion!

The LH and FSH cause your ovaries to "turn on." The ovaries then produce other hormones, primarily *estrogen* and *progesterone*. Estrogen and progesterone cause many of the physical changes you experience during puberty: breast development, widening hips, and *menstruation*, which is the monthly passage of blood and other tissues through the vagina. *Androgens*—the male sex hormones that all men and women produce—are responsible for further changes during puberty: growth spurts, acne, and the appearance of under-arm and pubic hair. Androgens come from the adrenal glands, which sit on top of each kidney.

Don't worry about memorizing these complicated terms. The most important thing is that you have a general idea of what's happening in your body. Just realizing that your body is undergoing a lot of changes will help you deal better with those changes.

Am I Normal?

As your body develops and your emotions seesaw, you may find yourself asking this question a million times: Am I normal? You wonder why your friend is a 32C while you are still flat, or why you go through 15 different emotions an hour while your best pal still seems like her same old self.

Relax. You *are* normal. It's just that puberty affects different girls in different ways. You may be an early bloomer or a late starter. You may feel like an emotional wreck or sail through puberty with barely a care. Basically, there is no such thing as normal!

Also keep in mind that as far as your body is concerned, everyone develops at her own speed. It may take some girls five or six years to go through puberty. Others may zip through it in two or three years. On the way toward fully developing, your body goes through many gradual changes, too. Some of these changes may be so gradual that you don't even notice that you're making progress!

If you feel that something is wrong, it's always best to check with a doctor. He or she can give you a thorough physical examination and reassure you that your body is on the right track—and moving along at the right speed for you.

CHAPTER 2

*Y*our Body's First Changes

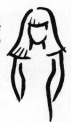

"Lately I'm afraid to wear a bathing suit. I'm younger than everyone in my class, and a lot of older kids don't have breasts yet. I do. I feel embarrassed, plus I don't want them to think I'm showing off."

—Tess Broach, age 9½, Sumner, Iowa

*H*ere are two of the first signs you're growing up: the appearance of breasts and pubic hair.

Your Changing Breasts

The physical change that is likely to make you feel more self-conscious than any other during puberty is your developing breasts, or in some cases, your lack of developing breasts. You may be worried that your breasts are never going to grow. Or, if your chest is bigger than most other girls', you may feel they're growing too quickly. And no matter what stage your breasts are in, you can't help but compare yourself with your girlfriends. You're also dying to know: *Do they or don't they wear bras yet?*

THE WAITING GAME

When can you expect your breasts to grow? Most girls' breasts begin to grow somewhere between the ages of 9 and 14. The process is gradual. It can take up to four or five years before your breasts reach their adult size.

BREAST DEVELOPMENT STAGES

There are five stages of breast development. They're called "Tanner stages," after the doctor who first described them.

Stage 1 (pre-puberty): Breasts are flat except for nipples.

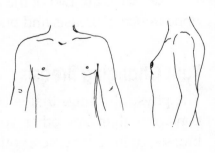

Stage 2 (puberty begins): The tissue under each nipple and the rest of the breast raise slightly, forming breast buds. The nipples also start to grow larger. The *areola*, the circle of skin surrounding each nipple, gets wider and darker.

Stage 3: The breasts and areolas become larger and blend into each other.

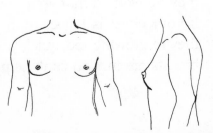

Stage 4: Each nipple and are-ola form a small, separate mound so that they stick out above the rest of the breast.

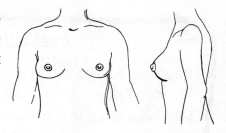

Stage 5: Breasts grow round and full. The nipples stick out, and the areola is no longer a raised mound on the breast.

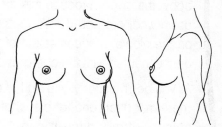

Not all girls go through every stage of breast development. Some go directly from Stage 3 to Stage 5, skipping Stage 4 altogether. Most girls start their periods somewhere during Stages 3 or 4 of breast development.

ALL SHAPES AND SIZES

You may start to worry when you notice your breasts don't look exactly like those of your friends or of your mother. For example, your breasts may be pointy, while your best pal's are round. You may already be filling a C cup and still have more growing ahead of you; a friend may stop for good at a B cup.

It's important to keep in mind that breasts come in all shapes and sizes. There is no one "right" shape, just as there is no one "right" size. So whatever you are, it's the right shape and size for you!

Your weight may also have something to do with your breast size. If you're super-skinny, your breasts may be smaller than average. Or, if you're a little pudgy, fatty tissue may increase the size of your breasts.

WHAT'S IN A BREAST?

Breasts are made up of some 15 to 20 different sections, called *lobes*. Each lobe is surrounded by a layer of fat.

Inside each lobe are structures called *alveoli*. When a woman has a baby, the alveoli produce milk for the baby to drink. The milk travels down what are called *milk ducts* to the nipple. When a baby sucks on the nipple, milk comes out of tiny openings in the nipple, which are connected with the openings of the milk ducts.

As you begin puberty, you start to develop milk ducts and fatty tissue. These milk ducts and fat are what form your breast buds. The development of milk ducts is one more way your body is readying itself for the time when (and if!) you decide to have a baby.

That's not all that's in a breast. Breasts also contain nerves, arteries, smaller blood vessels, lymph channels, and connective fibers to give breasts their final, rounded shape.

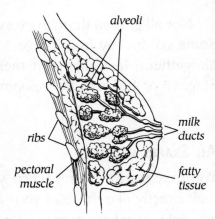

Cross Section of a Breast

Get These Questions Off Your Chest!

Q. *I'm 11 and still flat. I'm worried I won't get breasts until I'm 12 or 13. If my breasts don't start developing until I'm older, does that mean they won't grow as much?*

A. No. Your starting date has nothing to do with the ultimate size of your breasts. An early starter could end up with relatively small breasts, a late bloomer with large breasts.

Q. *I'm 13, and my breasts are pretty small. Can I do any exercises to make them larger?*

A. In your mom's and grandmother's time, girls used to practice arm and chest exercises, chanting, "I must, I must, I must increase my bust."

However, this exercise, and any others, won't increase the size of your breasts. Why? Because your breasts don't have any muscles, they won't grow as a result of exercise. You could do a thousand chest thrusts a day and your breasts would stay the exact same size! Stay away from any breast creams or bust-enhancement devices you may read about or see on TV ads, too!

There are, however, muscles on the chest wall just beneath your breasts called *pectoral* muscles. Developing these muscles may thicken the overall size or width of your chest, but it won't make your breasts bigger.

Q. *My areolas are pink. I thought they were supposed to be dark. Is something wrong?*

A. The areola ranges in color from light pink to dark brown. Sounds like you're perfectly normal!

Q. *My breasts are sore and tender to the touch. I'm worried that I've got some strange disease!*

A. Relax. While your breasts grow, a little soreness is normal. After all, your breasts are undergoing quite a big change. If, however, you are experiencing shooting pains; soreness accompanied by redness, warmth, or sudden swelling of the skin; a lump or hardness in the breast that wasn't there before; or any discharge from the nipple, check with your doctor just to be sure nothing is wrong.

Q. *One of my breasts is larger than the other. I've started walking with one shoulder hunched down so no one will notice. Will my other breast ever grow larger?*

A. Most likely, yes. It's very common for one breast to develop faster than the other. (And we bet that no one but you notices that your breasts are a tad uneven!)

In most cases, the smaller breast will eventually catch up with the other one. But keep in mind that most women's breasts do not match each other perfectly. Most women have one breast that is a little larger than the other. However, this difference is so tiny that no one else usually notices.

Q. *Help! I've started growing little hairs around my nipples. I've waited so long for breasts, and now they're hairy! What should I do?*

A. Believe it or not, many girls grow hair on their breasts. As long as it's just a few hairs, it's nothing to worry about. However, if you're really concerned with the way it looks, see your doctor. He or she may be able to recommend safe ways to remove the hair.

In the meantime, whatever you do, don't pluck the hairs out. This can lead to soreness and infection.

Q. *I know that nipples are supposed to stand out, but mine stick in instead. What's going on?*

A. You have what are called inverted nipples. Many girls and women have them.

Inverted nipples are nothing to be concerned about. The only time to worry about inverted nipples is if a nipple that wasn't inverted suddenly becomes so. If that happens, you should see a doctor just to make sure everything is okay.

Your First Bra

Do you need a bra? What size should you get? And will you live through the experience of having some fussy saleswoman tug and pull on you as she tries to find the "perfect fit"?

Figuring out if and when you need a bra is a major deal. Plus, you may feel embarrassed even thinking about bras, much less talking about them! This section will help alleviate your fears on the big "B" word!

WHO NEEDS A BRA?

If your breasts are starting to feel heavy and uncomfortable, you probably need a bra. Or maybe your mom will be the first one to point out that you could use a little support. Either way, feel free to talk about bras with your mom. She'll no doubt be able to help you feel comfortable with the idea, and she'll give you moral support as you go on your first bra-shopping spree!

If you really don't need a bra yet but feel left out because some of your friends are wearing them, you can buy a "training bra," a stretchable bra just for girls like you.

SIZING UP THE SITUATION

32A. 34C. 36DD. How does this weird way of measuring bra sizes work, anyway?

To get the right size of bra for you, you need to measure two different areas. The first measurement is chest size, which refers to how big around your chest is. That's why, when you go to buy a bra, the first thing the saleswoman will do is measure your chest size in inches. This number, such as 30, makes up the number part of the bra size.

The second measurement is cup size, and that measures how full your breasts are. The best way to figure out this size is to try on a few different bras and see which feels most comfortable for you. The most common cup sizes are A, B, and C.

- an A cup is for relatively small breasts

- a B cup is for medium-sized breasts

- a C cup is for full, rounded breasts

You can also find size AA bras for girls who are just beginning to develop, and size DD bras for girls with very large breasts.

Even if you think you know your size, make sure to try on several bras before choosing one because sizes and cup shapes differ from manufacturer to manufacturer. It also may help to have someone experienced in the dressing room to help you, but only if you feel comfortable with her.

Playing It Safe

Once you have breasts, you'll want to make sure they're healthy. One way to do this is to give yourself regular breast exams, first to become familiar with the feel of your breasts to know what normal is, and second to check for any lumps or other irregularities that could indicate breast cancer.

Most lumps or irregularities you find at your age are *not* cancer. But if you do find something, you must check with a doctor just to be safe.

There are two parts to the breast exam—*looking* at your breasts, then *feeling* them. For the visual part, you will need a mirror. There are several ways to do the manual part.

Visual Exam

Mirror, Mirror on the Wall

Turn on a bright light and step in front of a mirror. Then follow these steps:

1. Look carefully at each breast. Check for any bulge, depression, swelling, or patch of rough skin. Also check to see if your breasts have changed color anywhere.

2. Check out your nipples. Have they become inverted? Have the areolas changed color or do they feel different?

3. Take another look at your breasts with your hands clasped behind your head. Also look at your breasts with your hands pushing down on your hips. Sometimes lumps only show up when you are in these positions.

4. Gently squeeze each nipple to see if any fluid comes out. Fluid isn't necessarily a sign

that something's
wrong. However, if
your nipples are leak-
ing, see a doctor imme-
diately just to be safe.

MANUAL EXAM

Method 1: Sudsing Up in the Shower

Examining your breasts in the shower is a good idea because
your hands will slide easily over your body. Follow these steps:

1. With your fingers flat, place your left hand on the nipple
of your right breast. Extend your right arm straight up.
Imagine that your nipple is the center of a circle. With the
tips of your middle three
fingers, make tiny circular
movements, starting at
the nipple and moving
in a clockwise motion
around the breast.
(Another way of
doing this is to make
a small circle around
your nipple. Still using
the nipple as the center
of your circle, continue
to make larger and larger
circles, moving outward
toward the armpit. Either
method is fine, as long as
you cover the entire breast.) If you feel
any lump or abnormal swelling, check with your doctor.

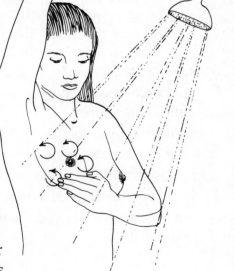

2. Feel under your arm as well, as some breast tissue reaches that far.

3. Repeat, using your right hand on your left breast.

Method 2: Lying Down

When following this method to examine your breasts, use a pillow to make it easier.

1. To examine your left breast, put a pillow under your left shoulder. This will help distribute the breast tissue evenly.

2. Place your left hand behind your head. Then, just as you did in the shower, make circles with your right hand around your left breast. (Again, you can either make tiny circular movements, moving in a clockwise motion around the breast, or make a small circle around the nipple, with the circles getting larger.) Be sure to cover your entire breast.

3. Repeat for your right breast.

It's best to examine your breasts once a month. A good time is right after your period. Before your period, your breasts may feel lumpy because of swelling of normal breast tissue due to hormonal changes. Make it a habit to begin with the visual exam, followed by either method of the manual exam.

Gone Yesterday, "Hair" Today

The other early telltale sign of puberty: You're growing pubic hair.

Now, pubic hair isn't exactly a subject you'd naturally sit down and chat about with your girlfriends. Sure, you may compare notes on other growing-up stuff, like how many pimples have popped up, but who wants to talk about pubic hair?

Of course, when you're alone, you no doubt check out this area of your body, searching for the latest strand and wondering if what's happening down there is normal.

We don't want you to waste any time worrying about what's going on. So here's how you can expect your pubic hair to grow.

Pubic Hair Development Stages

Pubic hair growth, just like breast growth, doesn't happen overnight. In fact, there are five different stages of pubic hair development.

Stage 1 (prepuberty): There is no pubic hair, except for possibly a few fuzzy or downy hairs.

Stage 2 (puberty begins): The first real hairs begin to grow. They are straight and fine, and slightly dark in color.

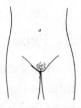

Stage 3: The pubic hair increases and gets thicker, coarser, and curlier. It may also get darker in color.

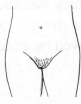

Stage 4: The pubic hair continues to get even thicker and curlier and to cover a larger area.

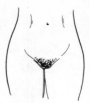

Stage 5: The hair is thick, coarse, and tightly curled: the pubic hair of an adult. It usually grows in an upside-down triangle. Sometimes the hair will continue to grow toward your belly button or down the insides of your thighs.

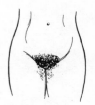

At what age will you start to grow pubic hair? Every girl is different, but in general, most girls reach Stage 3 of pubic hair development somewhere between the ages of 11 and 13. Most girls start their periods when they are at Stage 3 of pubic hair development.

Keep in mind that even when your pubic hair is all grown in, it may not look exactly like anyone else's. Some women have a lot of pubic hair; others have hair that's barely there. It may be blond, brown, black, or red. It may match the color of the hair on your head, or it may not.

It is important to keep the pubic area clean, just as you would the rest of your body. Suds up with whatever body soap you use and rinse well. This is especially important during menstruation, when blood may collect there.

ᕔ

WHAT'S IT FOR?

Pubic hair actually serves an important function. It helps keep the area between the outer lips of your vagina clean. Just like your eyelashes keep dust and other irritating particles from falling into your eyes, pubic hair protects this sensitive area from things that could irritate it.

CHAPTER 3

More Body Action

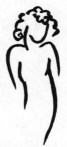

"My feet are a lot bigger now. They're a size 7½. I wish they were smaller. I'm taller too. A lot of boys are still shorter than me. But I only like the guys who are taller than me."

—Jonelle Dukes, age 12, East Rutherford, New Jersey

Besides developing breasts and pubic hair, your body changes in many other ways during puberty.

Hitting New Heights

Now that you're growing up, you're also growing taller.

Your favorite pair of jeans is turning into geeky highwaters. And your skirts are taking "mini" to a new level!

Not only that, parts of your body are growing more quickly than the rest. Your hands may suddenly grow, or maybe your feet. You may find your size 6 Keds to be crippling while your big brother's size 7 Reeboks fit like a charm.

If you're feeling a little gawky or out of proportion, don't worry. The rest of your body will catch up as you continue to go through puberty.

When can you expect to shoot up? While each girl is on her own timetable, most girls go through a growth spurt around the age of 11 or 12, right after their breasts have begun to develop.

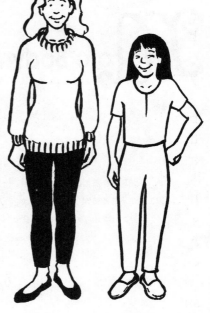

Once you start growing, you may be surprised at how quickly you grow. Before puberty, you gained an average of 2 inches of height a year. Now that you're entering puberty, you may grow as much as 6 inches in a year!

This period of quick growth starts to slow down as your body gears up for menstruation. By the time you start menstruating, you will have attained 90 to 95 percent of your adult height. You may expect to gain 2 or 3 more inches over the two years following menarche.

How tall will you end up being?

A lot of it depends on your heredity (traits you inherited from your parents). If your parents are tall, chances are you'll be tall yourself. If they're short, you may be on the shorter side, too. However, other factors come into play, so it's hard to predict.

Growing Pains

Your parents may complain that you're going through "growing pains," but most likely it's your occasional bratty behavior they're talking about, not your body!

However, right now you may actually be feeling some pains in your legs and other parts of your body called "growing pains." Doctors and researchers don't know exactly what causes growing pains. It is believed that most growing pains are probably muscle aches that kids your age get simply because you run around all day!

The most common places to feel growing pains are behind your knees, in front of your thighs, and along your shins.

You may also feel occasional twinges of pain in your arms, back, groin, or shoulders. Growing pains usually occur late in the day or during the night. They may even awaken you from a deep sleep.

Growing pains can be an annoying problem. Relieve the hurt by soaking in the tub, applying a warm compress, massaging your limbs, or taking a pain medication such as Acetominophen or Ibuprofen. (Before taking *any* medication, check with your parents.)

If the pains continue or worsen, see your doctor to make sure that your growing pains aren't actually a symptom of a more serious medical problem.

IF I'M SO TALL, WHY ARE ALL THE GUYS SO SHORT?

You may notice that while you and most of your friends have grown in height, most of the boys in your class haven't.

Why are they still *so short?*

Simply put, they probably haven't started puberty yet. Girls start puberty about two years before guys, so you have a few years growing time on them! But don't worry, the guys will soon catch up with you—even if you're the tallest girl in class.

Sweat It!

You used to tease your brothers about how gross they smelled after hours of sweaty football practice. Now, suddenly, you may be experiencing a few sweat stains yourself—on your favorite T-shirts, no less! To add insult to injury, you've taken a few whiffs of yourself lately, and, well . . . phew!

Welcome to the world of puberty and overactive sweat glands. The male sex hormones, androgens, turn on the sweat glands in all men and women during puberty. Once they're turned on, the perspiration that collects in body crevices can lead to body odor.

Luckily, you can arm yourself against a perspiration problem by doing the following:

> ### THE SHAPE OF THINGS TO COME
>
> During puberty, not only are you growing taller, you're filling out, too. Suddenly, you've got curves! Your hips are rounder, and so is your rear.
>
> Your face will probably start filling out as well.
>
> During puberty, female body weight increases about 10 to 20 percent (mostly due to an increase in body fat). Weight gain is completely normal and healthy, and it doesn't mean you need to lose weight. Girls who don't go through this change (because of excessive dieting or exercising, for example) often delay the onset of puberty and menstruation.

- Bathe or shower every day.
- After bathing, follow up by applying either a deodorant or antiperspirant.

What's the difference between a deodorant and an antiperspirant? The first covers up any odor from perspiration, while the second helps prevent you from perspiring in the first place. You can also find dual antiperspirants/deodorants on the market.

When applying either of these, wait until you've cooled down from the bath or shower. Also let the deodorant or anti-perspirant dry a little before putting on your clothes. Otherwise, you may be wearing as much on your shirt as under your arm!

If you're wearing an antiperspirant and start to sweat dur-ing the day, reapply it as needed.

Hair It Is

Another new development to watch for: hair under your arms. This generally happens sometime after your first period. Contrary to what you may have heard, it's not necessary to shave in order to cut down on underarm odor. Staying clean is more important. However, you may feel more comfortable shaving.

During puberty, the hair on your legs may also become darker and thicker. Deciding whether or not to remove this hair is also a personal decision. Some girls prefer the natural look, while others like a smoother look and feel.

Some women and girls also shave around their pubic hair area, removing only those hairs that are visible when they are wearing a bathing suit. You must be very careful when shav-ing in this sensitive area, because it often leads to irritation.

There are several ways to remove unwanted hair (as long as it's okay with your parents!). Most girls opt for shaving because it's the simplest and cheapest way to get rid of hair. An electric razor is easier to use, but a blade razor gives you the smoothest shave.

How can you make sure you don't end up looking like a victim of a slasher movie once you've got a blade razor in your hand? Read on for tips on shaving your legs, underarms, and pubic area:

- Soak your skin well in warm water before shaving (or shave after a bath or shower). That way, your skin will be softer and the hairs can be cut more easily.

- Shave in the direction the hair grows, not against it.

- On your legs, use long, slow strokes. Don't feel you're trying to beat the clock when you shave or you may end up with nicks and cuts. Pay special attention to the sensitive areas of the shin bone and knee.

- Use a moisturizer on your legs between shaves to cut down on skin dryness or irritation.

There are other ways to remove hair that use chemicals, wax, or electric currents. These can be irritating to the skin and need to be done with extra care or by a professional. For that reason, we recommend that for now, if you want to remove any unwanted hair, stick to shaving.

Breakout Bummer!

"Mom says I'll outgrow skin problems, but it seems like forever."
—Beezus Quimby in Beverly Cleary's *Ramona Forever*

The day you get your first pimple will go down as a black day in your diary. But remember, when a blemish rears its ugly head, you're not alone!

Practically every girl or boy who enters puberty is bound to battle the blemishes. Some have bad skin for only one or two years; others suffer from acne even into adulthood.

Why does puberty signal the start of acne attacks?

The oil glands in your skin become more active at that time. Most of these oil-producing glands are located on your face, chest, back, shoulders, and upper arms. This is why these parts of your body can be "hot spots" for acne.

The oil glands "pump" their oil into certain hollow hair shafts (or follicles) that end as little openings or pores on the surface of your skin. If these follicles get clogged with oil and skin cells, bacteria found on the skin's surface start to accumulate inside the follicle, causing the follicle to become infected. Soon, a pimple appears. If the opening of the follicle, or pore, closes over, a whitehead forms. If the top of the follicle remains open, a blackhead forms. (The black color is probably from pigmented skin cells.)

> ## COMPLEXION CULPRITS
>
> Acne can be caused by:
>
> - Oily makeup or moisturizers
> - Stress
> - Your period. When you menstruate, your sweat follicles become more narrow and so clog more easily.
> - Your heredity. If your parents had acne, there's a greater chance you will.
> - Sweating
> - Hair on the forehead. Hair contains dirt and oil that can clog pores.

Some people's follicles tend to clog more easily, and they are therefore more prone to developing pimples. Other people sail through adolescence with unclogged follicles and a clear complexion.

COMING CLEAN

While you may not be able to prevent acne, you can control it and treat it with proper skin care. Follow these healthy skin tips:

- Wash pimple-prone areas with warm water and a mild soap two to three times a day. If you can't get to a sink to suds up, use a non-oily cleansing lotion that you just smear on, then wipe off.

- If you have extra-oily skin, remove any excess oil after washing by dipping a cotton ball in an astringent and gently wiping the cotton ball over trouble spots.

- Blot any excess oil between washings by pressing a clean facial tissue to your face.

- Use only oil-free moisturizers for your face. Select noncomedogenic (non-acne-forming) makeup. (Makeup manufacturers will have this information on their product packaging.)

- Remove all makeup from your face each night.

- Keep your hair off your face.

- If more than a few pimples crop up, see your doctor. If necessary, he or she can give you prescription medications and treatments to help your skin, or can refer you to a skin doctor called a dermatologist for further treatment.

ACNE MYTHS

Before you start scrubbing your face with steel wool or vowing never to eat chocolate again to get rid of pesky pimples, check out the facts (and fiction!) of acne.

Myth #1: *Chocolate, as well as fried, fatty, and junk foods, cause acne.*

The Truth: There is no scientific evidence to support the notion that specific foods have an effect on skin.

Myth #2: *The quickest way to get rid of a pimple is to pop it.*
The Truth: Popping a pimple is the quickest way to *aggravate* acne. Popping, probing, or picking a pimple will only make it worse. It opens up the follicle and spreads the infection.

More important, a pimple today could become a scar tomorrow.

Myth #3: *A blackhead is caused by dirty pores.*
The Truth: A blackhead is a clogged follicle with its surface still open.

Myth #4: *The harder you scrub your face, the fewer pimples you'll get.*
The Truth: Scrub-a-dub-dubbing your face can cause almost as much damage as popping pimples. Rubbing your face too hard will only spread the infection.

Myth #5: *Soaking up the sun's rays will clear up your skin.*
The Truth: While some people's skin may be helped by a dry, warm climate, that's not true for everyone. Some people's acne actually gets worse in the summer, especially if they sweat a lot.

SAVE FACE!

Below are different specific treatments for treating acne. Consult a dermatologist before using any of these products to determine which one will be most effective and safest for you.

Product: Benzoyl Peroxide

This is the key ingredient in over-the-counter acne products such as Oxy 5 or Clearasil. It comes in different concentrations

(2.5 percent, 5 percent, 10 percent) and is available in creams, lotions, soaps, washes, or gels (the latter by prescription only).

Effectiveness

Benzoyl peroxide is a good first step, and it may be all you need to clear up mild acne. It works by helping to unclog the follicles. It also acts as an antibiotic, fighting the bacteria that cause blemishes.

How to Use

- Before using, test your sensitivity to the product by smearing some on your forearm and leaving it on for a few hours. If any rash develops, don't use the product. If the rash persists, call your doctor.

- Read all package directions carefully before using.

- Apply only a thin film.

- Start with the smallest concentration (2.5 percent) applied every other day, for several days. Then try daily use. Do the same if you begin using a 5 percent or 10 percent product, working up to daily use over the course of three to four weeks.

- Wait a few minutes after washing your face to apply. Moisture causes your face to absorb more of the product. This can irritate your skin. Be sure to cover all areas that might break out, not just areas already broken out.

Side Effects

- Can bleach your clothes.

- Can irritate skin. If redness or burning occurs, consult your doctor.

Product: Vitamin A Acid (Retin-A) (prescription only)

Effectiveness

Retin-A is more powerful than benzoyl peroxide. It not only helps to unplug follicles, but it also prevents them from clogging in the first place. Retin-A is not a quick cure. Your acne may even seem worse right after starting treatment, and it may take several months of use before you're likely to see results.

How to Use

- Follow your doctor's instructions.

Side Effects

- redness
- peeling
- dry skin

Product: Topical Antibiotics (prescription only)

Effectiveness

Topical antibiotics, such as Clindamycin, Erythromycin, and Tetracycline, stop the growth of the bacteria that contribute to acne.

How to Use

- Follow your doctor's instructions.

Side Effects

- dry skin
- discoloration of skin (Tetracycline only)
- skin fluoresces under black lights (Tetracycline only)

Product: Oral Antibiotics (prescription only)

Effectiveness

Your doctor may prescribe Tetracycline or Erythromycin in the form of a pill or liquid if topical medications aren't working.

How to Use

- Follow your doctor's instructions.

Side Effects

- nausea or upset stomach
- vaginal yeast infection
- diarrhea
- skin rashes

CHAPTER 4

Sexual Organs: The Simple Facts

"You wouldn't know a fallopian tube if you fell over one."
—Janie Gibbs to Harriet Welsch in Louise Fitzhugh's *The Long Secret*

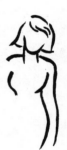

You are born with special sexual and reproductive organs both inside and outside your body. During puberty, these organs begin to grow and mature.

The *external female genitalia* are those sexual organs that you can see between your legs. The *internal genitalia* or reproductive organs are those inside your pelvis.

The Outside Story: External Female Genitalia

The best way to understand this area of your body is to pay close attention to the illustration on the next page. Or, if you feel comfortable with the idea, scoot yourself up to a mirror and look at your own genital area.

Most likely you haven't spent a lot of time looking "down there." The whole idea may make you squeamish, or you may feel embarrassed that you're even curious about that part of your body. But the more you know about your body, the more comfortable you'll feel living in it!

Here's what you'll see:

External Female Genitalia

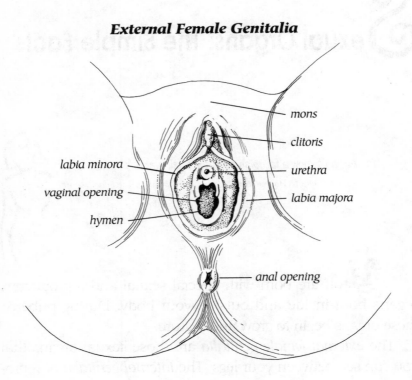

Vulva: The genital organs on the outside of a woman's body are referred to as the vulva. The vulva is made up of several parts:

Mons: This is a pad of fat tissue that covers the pubic bone. Pubic hair begins to grow on the mons during puberty. The mons also gets fleshier during puberty and starts to stick out more.

Outer Lips (or the labia majora): The vulva divides into two separate folds of skin, or "lips" (labia). These lips help protect the area underneath.

During puberty, pubic hair will begin to grow on them. The lips will also get fleshier and may begin to touch each other.

While the outer lips are smooth when you're a child, as you go through puberty, they may wrinkle. They tend to stay that way during most of your adult life.

Oil glands on the underside of the lips (these look and feel like small raised bumps) keep the area moist during puberty. So you may notice a little wetness that never used to be there before.

Inner Lips (or the labia minora): If you were to separate the outer lips, you would find an inner lip at either side of the opening of the vagina.

The skin covering them is pink, smooth, moist, and hairless. During puberty, the inner lips grow, but in general, they remain hidden by the outer lips. They may also become more wrinkled.

Clitoris: Near the top of the vulva where the inner lips meet is the clitoris. In some women, the lips come together, forming a "hood" for the clitoris, also known as the *prepuce*. The clitoris is very sensitive, and when it is touched, a woman may become sexually aroused.

Vaginal Opening: This opening is right below the urethra. It leads to the vagina, which is inside your body and can't be seen from the outside.

Hymen: The vaginal opening is covered by a thin piece of skin called the hymen. The hymen itself usually has an opening that enlarges as you grow.

Urethra: Technically not part of the external female genitalia, the urethra is nonetheless found in that area. It is the tiny opening just below the clitoris and just above the vaginal opening. Your urine passes through there.

The Inside Story:
Internal Genitalia (Reproductive Organs)

"I can name all the girl parts inside a woman's body because my mom just had a baby. I'm kinda embarrassed about knowing all that stuff. It seems like you shouldn't have to know about it until you're at least . . . 32!"

—Annie Wight, age 8, Centralia, Missouri

The sex organs or internal genitalia inside a woman's body are called reproductive organs because they are involved in reproducing (creating) babies. Here's what they do and how they work:

Internal Female Reproductive Organs

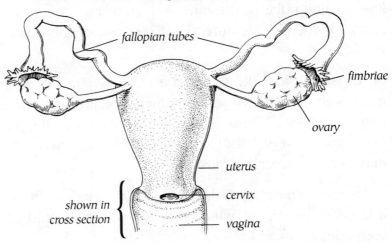

fallopian tubes

fimbriae

ovary

uterus

cervix

shown in cross section {

vagina

Vagina: The vagina is the stretchy, moist passageway that menstrual blood and tissue pass through.

It leads from the vaginal opening to the *cervix* (which you'll learn more about on page 44), which in turn leads to the uterus. During puberty, the vagina becomes longer.

Most of the time, the vagina is like a deflated balloon, with all of its inner walls touching. However, during sex, the vagina stretches to allow a man's penis to fit inside. And during childbirth, this small organ expands enough to allow a baby to pass through!

Once you begin puberty, you may feel some wetness in your vagina. The vagina contains glands that lubricate the area when you're feeling sexually excited. Even if you're not feeling sexually aroused, your vagina may be wet. This is because during puberty, under the influence of hormones, the walls of your vagina begin to shed their cells at a very fast rate, and the vagina produces fluid to wash these cells away. Other cells may also produce a mucous substance.

As you enter puberty, you may start to notice a clear or milky white, odorless watery discharge from your vagina that leaves a yellowish stain on your underpants. This increase in

Female Reproductive System
(cross section)

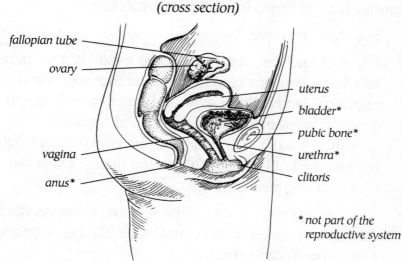

fallopian tube

ovary

uterus

bladder*

pubic bone*

vagina

urethra*

clitoris

anus*

** not part of the
reproductive system*

vaginal discharge may begin several months to a year before the onset of menstruation.

Once you begin menstruating, this discharge may change from sticky to stringy and slippery (like egg whites) as you near ovulation. Don't worry— it may sound strange, but it's perfectly normal!

Cervix: If you were to put a finger into your vagina and reach all the way in, you'd feel a round knob that feels like the tip of your nose. (By the way, it's perfectly safe to gently insert a clean finger into your vagina.)

In the center of your cervix is a small hole known as the *os.* Once you start your period, the menstrual flow passes through the os to the vagina and out of your body. When a woman is pregnant and about to give birth, this tiny opening also stretches wide enough for a baby to pass through.

Uterus: As you may already know, this is where a baby grows. Normally, the uterus is shaped like an upside-down pear, and it is empty. But during pregnancy, when it holds the growing baby, it expands to many times its size.

The uterus has three layers:

- The *endometrium,* which lines the inside of the uterus. This lining contains blood vessels (arteries and veins) and secretory glands. These grow and multiply each month to make the inside of the uterus spongy and cushiony.

  When a woman is pregnant, the endometrium helps nourish the baby growing inside the uterus. Otherwise, it is shed during menstruation.

- The *myometrium,* the coat of muscle that contracts during menstruation to expel blood and tissue. During pregnancy, it helps push out the baby.

- The *serosa,* the smooth outer covering of the uterus.

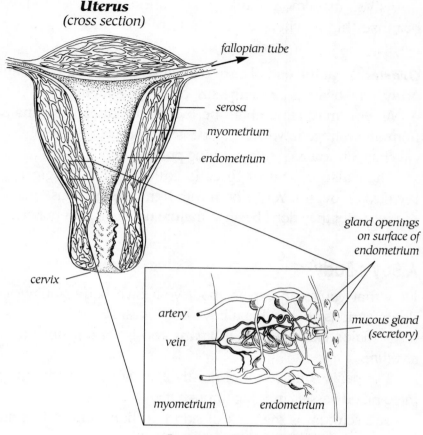

Uterus
(cross section)

fallopian tube

serosa

myometrium

endometrium

gland openings
on surface of
endometrium

cervix

artery

vein

mucous gland
(secretory)

myometrium   endometrium

Close-up of Endometrium

Fallopian Tubes (or uterine tubes): The fallopian tubes
extend from the top of the uterus. The ends of the tubes are
widened and frayed, like gloves flapping in the breeze. Each
tube is divided into many tentaclelike structures called *fimbriae.* When you ovulate each month, the fimbriae guide the egg
from an ovary into the fallopian tube.

Inside the fallopian tubes, the walls are lined with tiny
hairs called *cilia.* The cilia help to direct an egg from the tube
into the uterus. Contraction of the tube also helps move the
egg along.

As you may know, the fallopian tubes are very important because this is where an egg is fertilized, and pregnancy begins.

Ovaries: Near the end of each of the two fallopian tubes is an *ovary*. One ovary is about the size of a large almond.

As you may remember, the ovaries produce the female hormone estrogen, which is responsible for most of the physical changes you go through during puberty.

They also contain egg cells called *ova* (a single egg is called an ovum). You're born with hundreds of thousands of egg cells. But they don't begin to mature until you start puberty.

A Boy's Body

Now that you're an expert about your own body, you're no doubt curious about what a boy's body is all about.

A male's external sexual organs consist of a *penis* and a *scrotum*.

The penis is made up of mostly spongy tissue with many large blood vessels running through it.

The scrotum is the sack of skin that hangs down behind the penis and holds a boy's *testicles*. The testicles are two small egg-shaped organs, one inside each compartment of the scrotum. The left scrotum usually hangs lower than the right. The testicles are where sperm are made. These organs also contain cells that secrete the male sex hormone, *testosterone*. This is the hormone responsible for most of the sexual changes that occur in boys during puberty.

Normally, the penis hangs loose. However, when a man becomes sexually excited, the blood vessels inside the penis fill with blood. The penis swells, getting hard and erect. This is called an *erection*.

Boys have erections from the time they're born. Even baby

boys have them! However, when a boy enters puberty, it happens more often. A boy can have an erection just thinking about kissing and making out or by seeing a pretty girl.

A boy can even get an erection when he's not thinking about sex, like when he's watching a baseball game or lying out in the sun relaxing on a warm summer's day. He can also get one in the middle of the night while sleeping, or wake up with an erection.

An erection goes away either by itself, or through what's called an *ejaculation*. This is when a man has a sexual climax and whitish liquid spurts from the end of his penis.

This liquid is called *semen,* or *seminal fluid.* Semen is made up mostly of sperm cells transported in a mucous liquid. Semen comes out of the tip of the penis. Both urine and semen pass through the same opening—but not at the same time.

Male Reproductive System
(cross section)

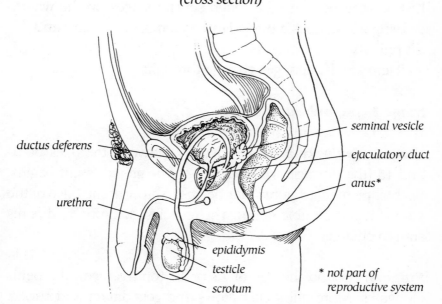

ductus deferens

urethra

seminal vesicle

ejaculatory duct

anus*

epididymis

testicle

scrotum

* not part of reproductive system

Where does semen come from?

Sperm cells are produced in the testicles. They pass from each testicle into the *epididymis,* the half-moon-shaped structure that sits directly on top of the testicle inside the scrotum. The sperm mature and are stored in the epididymis, where they are mixed with a mucous substance until they are emitted. The *ductus deferens* (also called the *vas deferens*) is a thin tube that carries the sperm from the epididymis down to the *ejaculatory duct.* The ejaculatory duct is located inside the body in the pelvic area. This ejaculatory duct receives not only the sperm, but also more fluid from a special gland called the *seminal vesicle.* Once the sperm are mixed with this fluid, the semen is propelled out into the *urethra* (which is a hollow tube that runs from the bladder, then along the entire length of the penis), and finally out of the penile opening during ejaculation.

HOW A BOY'S BODY DEVELOPS

Just as your body goes through several stages on the way to growing up, so does a boy's. However, most boys start and finish puberty later than girls.

Here are the changes guys go through:

Stage 1 (pre-puberty)

Stage 2 (puberty begins):
Usually between the ages of 10 and 15 (the average age is 12 or 13), the growth spurt begins. Slightly pigmented pubic hair begins to grow at the base of the penis (over the pubic bone). The testicles, scrotum, and penis start to enlarge.

Stage 3:
Around the age of 13 or 14 (on average), the penis elongates. More pubic hair grows and gets darker and curlier.

Underarm hair and facial hair appear. The testicles and scrotum continue to grow; sperm are made. The first ejaculation often occurs during this stage.

Stage 4: Around ages 14 to 16 (on average), the pubic hair gets coarser, and the facial and underarm hair continue to grow. The body is still gaining height and is now adding muscle mass. The first trace of a mustache is found. Acne and body odor occur for the first time. The boy's voice deepens. The scrotum, testicles, and penis continue to grow.

Stage 5: By the age of 17 or 18 (again, on average) the boy is now physically an adult. He has reached his full height, his genitalia has reached its full size, and he has developed his deepest voice. His body hair distribution is that of an adult, with pubic hair on the inner thighs and extending upward onto his abdomen.

CHAPTER 5

The "M" Word: Menstruation

"*Each time I have a period—and that has only been three times—I have the feeling that in spite of all the pain, unpleasantness, and nastiness, I have a sweet secret, and that is why, although it is nothing but a nuisance to me in a way, I always long for the time that I shall feel that secret within me again.*"

— Anne Frank, *The Diary of a Young Girl*

*O*f all the changes you're going through right now, the biggest one of all is starting your period. Once you start menstruating, you're officially on your way to becoming a woman.

Did You Hear the One About . . . ?

A funny thing happens the minute you start your period. You also start getting a lot of advice—from everyone from your best girlfriend to your great-aunt Matilda to the nosy next-door neighbor. While everyone means well, their advice can be as old-fashioned as the music your grandparents listen to!

How do you know what to tune out? By tuning in to some of the biggest myths about menstruation.

Myth #1: *Get lots of bed rest. In your "condition," you're too weak to be as active as you usually are.*

The Truth: Your period doesn't have to interfere with your normal life. In fact, the more active you are, the less likely you are to experience painful menstrual cramps and the better you'll probably feel.

Bopping with your pals to some tunes or challenging Dad to a game of tennis can help ease many of the painful symptoms that come along with your period.

Myth #2: *Run for cover when you see boys! If you get too close to them, they'll know you've got your period. How embarrassing!*

The Truth: Unless a guy has X-ray vision or you ask him for a tampon, he won't ever know you're menstruating. There are no special "Hey, I've got my period" vibes a girl sends out.

So relax, be yourself, and know that your secret is safe. Besides, as you get older, you'll quit worrying about whether or not guys know you have your period (you'll be certain they don't know!).

Myth #3: *Don't touch any houseplants. They'll die at your touch!*

The Truth: This old wives' tale is left over from centuries ago when menstruating women were thought to be dangerous. According to legend, they could cause milk to sour and wine to turn to vinegar.

Obviously, there's not one stitch of truth to this idea. So don't use it as an excuse to get out of your weekly plant-watering chores!

Myth #4: *Ban all baths. They aren't sanitary.*

The Truth: There's nothing unclean about taking baths. Soak away for as long as you like. In fact, it's essential that you bathe or shower on days when you have your period to keep clean and fight odor.

Myth #5: *Whatever you do, don't go swimming. That's not sanitary, either.*

The Truth: When you have your period, you can swim all you want. Just put in a tampon and dive in! (Don't swim with a sanitary pad on, because the pad will immediately absorb the water, not the blood.)

Myth #6: *Kiss your favorite animal three times at midnight each night you have your period, or you'll never get married.*

The Truth: Okay, okay, we made this one up. But it shows you just how far-out some of these myths are. (Besides, it never hurts to kiss your favorite stuffed animal.)

The point is, if someone tells you something about your period that's silly, confusing, or scary, consult your doctor. He or she will set you straight.

Why Do You Get Your Period?

The female body is designed to conceive and carry children. Your period is a signal that your body is probably able to get pregnant and have a baby.

THE MENSTRUAL CYCLE

Now we know what follows sounds pretty technical, but hang in there. It's actually pretty interesting stuff. You already learned some of these terms in Chapter 1. But for easy reference, we're also including them here.

So here's how your period works.

Every month, the pituitary gland in your brain releases a hormone called the follicle stimulating hormone (FSH). FSH chemically signals the eggs inside your ovaries to grow.

Each egg, or ovum, is inside its own protective "pod." This is called a *follicle* (which is how FSH got its name!). Every month one of the eggs develops more than the rest. Once an egg is fully developed, the pituitary gland receives a signal to release a second hormone called the luteinizing hormone (LH). This hormone causes the egg to be released from the surface of the ovary. This process is called *ovulation*. (The mound or clump of yellow tissue that remains at the site of the empty follicle is called the *corpus luteum,* which is how LH got its name.)

Menstrual Cycle

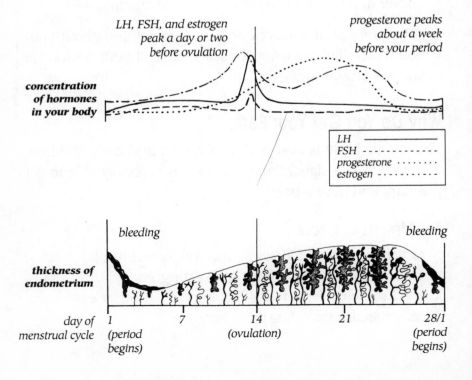

LH, FSH, and estrogen peak a day or two before ovulation

progesterone peaks about a week before your period

concentration of hormones in your body

LH ————————
FSH - - - - - - - - - - -
progesterone · · · · · · · ·
estrogen - · - · - · - · - ·

bleeding

bleeding

thickness of endometrium

day of menstrual cycle

1
(period begins)

7

14
(ovulation)

21

28/1
(period begins)

At the same time an egg is growing (before ovulation), FSH also causes the ovarian follicle to produce the hormone estrogen. Estrogen prepares the uterus each month for a possible pregnancy. It causes the lining of the uterus to become thick with soft cushiony tissue and new blood vessels.

Once ovulation occurs, the corpus luteum secretes another hormone, progesterone. Progesterone makes the lining of the uterus even thicker, filling it with larger blood vessels and nutrients, all to protect and feed a developing child.

What happens to the egg once it's released from the ovary? It heads for the uterus by way of one of the two fallopian tubes.

WHAT CAN YOU EXPECT DURING YOUR FIRST PERIOD?

The onset of your menstrual cycle is called *menarche*. The first time you menstruate, you probably won't leak much blood at all. Most girls start with just a few spots of bright red blood or a brown, sticky stain on their underpants.

So if you are caught unaware without a pad or tampon that very first time, you may be uncomfortable, but you probably won't have to worry about blood soaking through your clothes.

If, while the egg is in the fallopian tube, it meets and joins a male sperm (a process called *fertilization*), pregnancy begins. The fertilized egg takes a few days to complete its journey to the uterus and settle itself in the uterine lining. During pregnancy, the corpus luteum continues to make progesterone to keep the uterine lining healthy. (A hormone from the lining of the pregnant uterus itself stimulates the corpus luteum to keep producing the progesterone.)

If an egg is not fertilized by a sperm within 24 to 48 hours after it is released, it will disintegrate. The corpus luteum will disintegrate, too. Estrogen and progesterone levels fall, and the lining of the uterus breaks apart. A mixture of blood and tissue then exits your body through your vagina. When that happens, your menstrual flow, or period, has begun. You have also begun a brand new *menstrual cycle.*

Soon after your period is over, the whole process begins again, eventually resulting in your next period.

How Long Is a Menstrual Cycle?

Although the length of one cycle can last anywhere from 21 to 45 days, 28 days is the average. Don't be alarmed if your cycle lasts a little shorter or longer. Everyone's cycle length is different.

When you first begin your period, be prepared for a few irregularities in timing, duration, and flow. When you're first getting started, it's not uncommon to get your period once every two weeks or just once every few months.

Once your body gets the hang of the process (which may take a year or even two), you'll no doubt become more regular. The older you are when you get your first period, the longer it may take to become regular.

How Long Does a Period Last?

The length of a period differs for everyone, but in general, a period lasts between two and seven days. Five days is average. From month to month, the length of flow may vary.

How much flow there is also varies from girl to girl. You may start out with a light flow of blood and end up with a heavy flow, or vice-versa. You may also pass clots of blood and tissue, which is completely normal.

How much blood can you expect to lose? While you're menstruating, it can look like you're losing half your body's supply! But in most cases, you're only losing a very small amount—at most only about a quarter to a half cup. This amount is tiny when compared to your body's total blood supply.

If you find yourself soaking through four or five pads or tampons a day, consult a doctor. While there's probably no problem, it's best to get checked out if your flow is extremely heavy.

KEEPING TRACK

Once you're pretty regular, it's a good idea to chart your periods on a calendar. That way you can be prepared if your period starts when you least want it to—like when you're wearing a white skirt!

By marking down the first day of each period on a calendar and counting the days between periods, you'll probably begin to see a pattern.

Let's say that there are 30 days between the starting days of your periods. That means you're on a 30-day schedule. You should then be able to look ahead to the future and figure out about which day your period will next start.

Waiting for the Big Day

What if all of your pals have started their periods and you're feeling like the last girl on earth who hasn't? Relax. Your time will come. Most girls begin their periods between the ages of 10 and 16. The average age is 12½ years.

When you begin menstruating depends on a few different factors. Ask your mom how old she was when she started her period. Most girls menstruate around the same time their mothers did. So, if Mom had to wait until she was 15, you may be waiting that long, too!

Your body is also giving you clues as to when you'll start. Most girls begin their periods one or two years after their breasts have started developing. (Of course, there are no hard-and-fast rules. Some girls wait three years.)

If you are an athlete or very active physically, or if you are dieting and have experienced significant weight loss, your body may also put off menstruating. That's because the onset of puberty itself is delayed. Doctors are not sure why such delays happen. It's possible that a girl simply doesn't yet have enough body fat for puberty (and menarche) to begin.

CAN YOU GET PREGNANT BEFORE YOUR FIRST PERIOD?

Have you heard you can't get pregnant if you haven't had your period yet? Not true!

All it takes to get pregnant is for an egg to join with a sperm. And some girls ovulate (release an egg from an ovary) before they get their first period.

While it's much more common for girls to get their period a few times before they actually ovulate, some ovulate right from the beginning. If a girl has sex while she's ovulating, before she has ever had a period, she *can* get pregnant.

If you have any questions about when you're going to start, see your doctor. He or she can tell you what's normal for you.

Not Waiting?

"My mom has told me all about getting your period. It doesn't sound scary, because it's natural. But I'm not really looking forward to it. I hope I get it when I'm 13 or older."

—Amie Ray, age 10½, Los Angeles, California

What if your period is near, but you'd rather do 30 chores around the house than go through all of the emotional and physical changes that come with the start of your period?

If this is the case, share your feelings with your mom or another trusted adult. She or he will be able to reassure you.

You can also talk with friends who have already started their periods. The good thing about menstruation is that you never have to face it alone!

Now-You-See-'Em, Now-You-Don't Periods

Sometimes periods do a disappearing act. You may have had several normal, seemingly regular periods, then suddenly they stop for three or four months.

This condition has a fancy name called *secondary amenorrhea*. Why does this occur? There are many possible reasons:

- Pregnancy. If you are sexually active and have missed even one period, you should go to a doctor to make sure you aren't pregnant, even if you have only had your period for a few months.

- Stress. A tough test, a big blowout with Mom or Dad, or any other stressful situation can cause you to stop menstruating.

- Extreme weight loss or dieting

- Excessive weight gain

- Overexercising

- Long-term physical illness

- Some prescribed medications or illegal drugs

- Sudden changes in environment, like a long trip

- Hormonal problems

If you miss a period, check with your doctor. He or she will be able to pinpoint why your periods have stopped.

Cramp City!

Many girls and women experience cramps during their periods. They can be fairly mild, or they can be very painful. If painful enough, they sometimes can cause a girl to feel nauseated and throw up. Cramps also sometimes last an entire period. Other times they happen only at the start of a period.

What causes cramps? Most experts believe they're caused by hormonelike chemicals in your body that are called *prostaglandins*.

Prostaglandins cause the muscle in your uterus to contract during your period. The muscle contractions help the uterus expel the blood and tissue that line it.

> **WATCH THAT PAIN!**
>
> Some painful periods may be associated with other, more severe conditions. For this reason, if you have severe pain during a period, make sure to see a doctor.

While these contractions help perform an important function, they can also make you feel pretty darn miserable!

How to combat cramps? Here are some suggestions:

- Relax! It can help to lie down for a half hour with a heating pad (set on low) resting on your lower abdomen. A soothing bath can also make you feel better.

- Find relief by taking an over-the-counter, aspirin-free pain reliever—if it's okay with your doctor. (Ibuprofen is one of the most effective medications available.)

  For faster pain relief, take the medication at the first signs of pain. But make sure to take only the dosage prescribed on the back of the bottle.

- Often the best cramp buster of all is working out. So don't say no when your pals call to invite you on a bike ride by the beach or lake. Pack some healthy snacks, put on your bike shorts, and join your buddies. You're almost guaranteed to feel better getting fresh air and exercise than sitting inside thinking about how rotten you feel!

If none of these remedies helps your cramps, see a doctor. She or he may be able to prescribe medication to ease the pain.

Unfortunately, cramps aren't the only painful part of your period. You may also feel really tired and lethargic. Some girls get headaches or pains in their thighs, back, and groin. Just in case you're wondering, there's a technical term for all of these symptoms. It's called *dysmenorrhea,* or in plain language, painful periods.

Premenstrual Syndrome

You may have already heard your mom or other adult women in your life talk about premenstrual syndrome, otherwise known as PMS.

Some women suffer from one or many uncomfortable physical or emotional symptoms a week or two before their periods. These symptoms usually disappear on the first or second day of their periods.

If you have PMS, some of the symptoms you may feel before each period are:

- enlarged, tender breasts
- abdominal bloating (you can't zip those skintight jeans like you usually can!)
- backaches
- headaches

- increase or decrease in appetite

- cravings for salty or sweet foods

- constipation

- sore muscles

- fatigue

- increased need to urinate

- weight gain (just a pound or two)

- puffy hands or feet

- mood swings (anxiety, tension, depression)

Whew! That's a long list. But keep in mind that, if you develop PMS, it's likely you won't suffer from more than a few of these symptoms at any given time. More good news: Girls and women who suffer from PMS tend to have painless periods.

Since the causes of PMS are completely unknown, the treatment (at least for now) consists of using some common sense:

- Reduce your salt intake. Salt makes your body hold water. This can cause stomach bloating, puffiness, and weight gain.

  Say good-bye to foods such as chips, pretzels, bacon, cold cuts, diet sodas, and nuts for the week or two before your period (and during your period).

- Cut out sugary junk foods such as cookies, doughnuts, and cake a week or two before your period. All that sugar gives you a quick high, but then leaves you feeling more tired than before.

- Decrease or eliminate foods containing caffeine (sodas, chocolate, coffee, tea).

- Eat three well-balanced meals a day. Some girls leave

themselves open to premenstrual headaches because they simply don't eat enough. You may think not eating will eliminate any bloating or weight gain, but it won't.

- Exercise regularly. Working out helps not only cramps, but PMS as well.

If the above suggestions are not helping, you may have a severe case of PMS. Call your doctor immediately. She or he may be able to give you a strict diet to follow, or if necessary, some medication.

The Great Tampon Debate

Once you start your period, you've got a big decision in front of you. Do you use tampons or pads? And then there's the agony of buying them—pulling them off the shelves, throwing them casually in your grocery basket (covering them up with a big box of cereal), and hoping the checker doesn't notice your strawberry-red face when he or she rings the purchase up.

Deciding which to use—tampons or pads—is very personal. What's right for you may not be right for a friend. You may also hear some weird things about either method, such as you can't use a tampon if you're a virgin (which isn't true). Ignore these old wives' tales!

Give yourself some time to figure out which feels most comfortable for you before making any decision. And remember, no matter how embarrassed you are when you buy your first box of tampons or pads, you'll soon get over it. Before you know it, buying them will be as easy as picking out a pair of socks!

The following information will help you in making that "big decision."

SANITARY PADS

A sanitary pad is made of layers of soft, absorbent material with adhesive backing that sticks to your underwear.

It used to be that a woman's only option was to attach a sanitary napkin to a belt, and wear the belt around her waist. (Ask your mom about this!) The new adhesive pads are much more convenient and easier to wear.

Pads come in all different sizes, shapes, and absorbencies. If you have a heavy menstrual flow, you may need the thickest pad on the market. These are usually called super- or maxi-pads.

If your flow is on the light side, you'll probably be fine with a thinner pad or even an ultra-light one known as the mini-pad. For those days when you expect to get your period, you may want to wear a panty shield or liner for just-in-case protection.

When you first wear a pad, especially a thick one, you may feel a little bulky. But you'll get used to the feeling. You may also feel like everyone can tell you're wearing one—as if pads could somehow glow through your clothes! But rest assured that a pad doesn't show, no matter how bulky you may feel.

Change your pad about every three to four hours. If you flow heavily, you may need to change it more often. Sometimes a pad may smell if it's worn too long. While menstrual blood is clean and odorless, once it hits the air, it can smell a little.

When disposing a pad, do not flush it down a toilet. Wrap it up in toilet paper and put it in the trash can. The toilet paper will keep any odor under wraps.

TAMPONS

A tampon is a rolled cylinder of cotton and other material that you insert into the vagina to catch the menstrual flow. It has a string attached to the end of it, which hangs outside your vagina. When you need to remove the tampon, you simply pull on the string.

Like pads, tampons also come in a variety of absorbencies and sizes, from slender sizes for light-flow days to super sizes for days when you're flowing heavily.

You may worry that you'll never be able to put in a tampon. But once you get the hang of it, it's a cinch!

Keep in mind that tampons aren't for every girl. Some girls never feel comfortable using them. And, some doctors recommend that young girls shouldn't use tampons at all for the first two years after starting their periods due to the possibility of *toxic shock syndrome* (discussed on page 68). Before using tampons, check with your doctor to see what she or he recommends.

If you're sure you're ready to start using tampons, here are some simple steps to help you out:

PRACTICE DOESN'T MAKE PERFECT

It's okay to be eager to start using tampons. But don't practice inserting them *unless you have your period*. You see, when the tampon is soaked with blood, it will glide smoothly out of the vagina, but if it's dry, it will be very painful to pull out.

- Start out with the most slender tampon, as this will be the easiest to insert. The tampon should also come with an applicator, which makes the insertion process easier.

- Wash your hands thoroughly.

- Remove the outer wrapping. With your fingers, open the outer and inner lips covering the vagina, and put the tampon up to the vaginal opening.

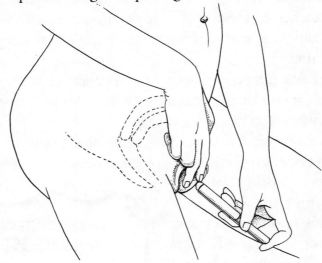

- Push the end of the tampon with the outer tube (not the end with the string!) into your vagina. Make sure to insert the tampon at a slight angle, as the vagina angles toward the small of the back.

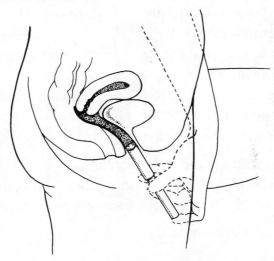

- Push the inner tube of the applicator into the outer tube. This will push the tampon itself farther into your vagina and out of the applicator. The applicator can then be removed and thrown away in the trash can.

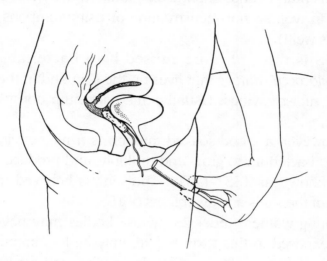

Make sure that the tampon goes high enough into your vagina. Otherwise it will feel uncomfortable or even painful. If a tampon is inserted correctly, you shouldn't feel it at all.

You can insert a tampon either standing, sitting, or lying down. After a bit of experimenting, you'll find which way feels most comfortable to you.

It's best to change a tampon every three to four hours to make sure you're not leaking and to stop any odors from developing.

If you're having trouble putting in a tampon, you may want to ask your doctor or other trusted adult about it. Chances are, you're inserting the tampon incorrectly and just need some practice.

After using a tampon, check the tampon box to see if it's flushable. If it's not, wrap it up in toilet paper and put it in the trash can.

Toxic Shock Syndrome

You've probably heard about toxic shock syndrome, otherwise known as TSS. This is a rare disease that has been linked to menstruation and, in particular, tampon use. (TSS can also occur in women not menstruating or using tampons and in men as well!)

TSS is thought to be caused by a bacterium called *Staphylococcus aureus* that lives on the skin and in the body's warm, moist cavities. Usually, this bacterium doesn't cause problems.

However, a blood-soaked tampon is a nice environment for this bacterium to grow and multiply, and produce a nasty toxin known as TSST-1. This "poison" is believed to cause many of the signs and symptoms of TSS.

Young women under 25, whose bodies may never have been exposed to this toxin before, may be less immune to it and therefore more likely to develop toxic shock syndrome.

TSS usually starts with a sudden high fever, followed by vomiting, diarrhea, light-headedness, achy muscles, headache, red eyes, and a sunburnlike rash, especially on the torso and thighs.

If you are using tampons and you develop any of these symptoms, see a doctor immediately. If left untreated, TSS can be fatal.

Safety Tips

- Change your tampon every three to four hours.
- Avoid super- or high-absorbency tampons.
- Never keep a tampon in overnight (use a pad).

Tampon Q&A: What If...? _____

Q. *Once a tampon is in, can it fall out? That would be pretty embarrassing!*

A. Luckily, that's something you won't ever have to worry about. The muscles inside your vagina hold the tampon tightly in place and prevent it from slipping out.

Q. *I want to start using tampons, but I've heard that sometimes a tampon can get lost up there and disappear into your body. Is this true?*

A. No. It's impossible for a tampon to get "lost." While it fits easily into your vagina, it is too big to go any farther.

It is blocked by the cervical canal, which is the passageway between the vagina and the uterus. The opening of the cervical canal is no bigger than the head of a match, and it's impossible for a tampon to get through.

Sometimes it may feel like the tampon is "lost" if the string attached to the end of the tampon somehow gets drawn up into the vagina. If this happens, just reach up inside and pull the tampon out with your fingers.

While a tampon can't get lost, keep in mind that a piece of material from a tampon may come off and stay in your vagina. This can lead to infection. If you experience any abnormal discharge after tampon use, see your doctor.

Q. *I've heard that some girls can't use tampons. They're just "too small." I'm scared I might be one of them because once, when I tried to put in a tampon, I couldn't get it in.*

A. Don't worry. You *can* use a tampon!

What's probably happening is that you're a little nervous about inserting a tampon, and your vaginal muscles are tightening up and making the vaginal opening smaller.

The next time you try to insert a tampon, relax. If the vaginal opening is dry, try lubricating the area with a little petroleum jelly.

You may also want to stretch the vaginal opening a little bit with your fingers. This may help you slip in a tampon more easily.

CHAPTER 6

What You Should Know About Sex

"My parents and I haven't talked about sex yet. I don't really want to yet. But I will soon. I think in a couple of months, I'll be ready to talk about it."

—Lauren Regan, age 10, Manassas, Virginia

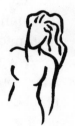

You may not think this chapter's for you.

Maybe you think you know everything already. Your parents have told you some facts of life. The rest you picked up from kids at school.

Or maybe you know just a little bit about sex, and you're not sure you want to know any more! After all, you're only a preteen. You're too young to care about all that sex stuff!

But no matter how little or how much you already know, it never hurts to learn more (besides, we bet you really don't know everything!).

The more you learn now, the better you'll be able to make smart decisions about sex as you grow up. This chapter covers some of the basics on sex, but your best source for answering all your questions (especially the more personal ones!) is your parents.

So That's What Happens . . .

Here's exactly what a couple does when they "do it":

When a man and woman care about each other, they may decide to have intercourse. They kiss and touch each other, becoming sexually aroused. When the man gets aroused, his penis becomes hard. The woman's vagina, when sexually excited, secretes a lubricating fluid inside the vagina. When the man puts his penis in a woman's vagina and moves it rhythmically inside, this is called sexual intercourse.

A woman can reach orgasm—the peak of sexual pleasure—once or several times during intercourse. When the man reaches an orgasm, he ejaculates semen into the woman's vagina. If one of the sperm in the semen meets and joins with an egg in the woman's body, she will become pregnant.

MILLIONS AND MILLIONS

Semen contains millions and millions of sperm. In fact, a normal ejaculation produces more than 300 million sperm. These sperm are so tiny that together they could *all* fit on the head of a pin.

Each sperm has three parts:

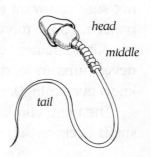

head

middle

tail

- the head, which contains the genetic material that the man contributes to making a baby

- the middle section, which gives the sperm the energy to move

- the tail, which propels the sperm forward

A man can produce the sperm needed to make a baby anytime. But as you know, a woman produces the egg that is needed only once a month. Pregnancy is most likely to occur if a couple has unprotected sex a few days before the woman ovulates or up to two days afterward.

How Life Begins

Each sperm contains 23 chromosomes, the genetic matter the father contributes to the baby. The woman's egg also has 23 chromosomes, the genetic matter the mother contributes to the baby.

After entering a woman's vagina, the sperm have one function: to find the woman's egg, which is resting in one of her fallopian tubes. The first sperm to completely penetrate the egg fertilizes it. (The fertilized egg is called a *zygote*.) After the

---

TWIN TALK

You probably know at least one set of twins, or you may even be a twin. How does this happen?

There are two types of twins, fraternal and identical. Fraternal twins occur if the mother produces two eggs instead of just one. Two separate sperm fertilize each egg. Fraternal twins are just as different from each other as any brother or sister are.

Identical twins are caused when a single fertilized egg (or zygote) splits into two parts (or three parts, for triplets!). Two fetuses develop, each containing the exact same genetic makeup. Identical twins will always be the same sex and look exactly alike (at least initially).

sperm penetrates the outer covering of the egg, the 23 chromosomes in both the sperm and egg are eventually united. Once the egg is fertilized, no other sperm can penetrate it.

The sperm's mission may sound easy, but it's actually very hard. The journey from the vagina to the fallopian tube is confusing. It's easy for the sperm to get "lost" and swim in the wrong direction. Some sperm are slow swimmers and simply die of "old age" before reaching their goal (a sperm can stay alive within a woman's body for only about 48 hours). Others are killed off as they pass through the cervical mucus.

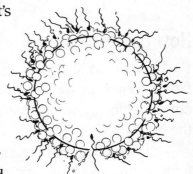

During fertilization, only 1 sperm makes it all the way inside the egg.

Birth Control

As you can see, sperm are very determined. They have one job: to go with the flow, find the egg, and fertilize it. Therefore, if you don't want to become pregnant, you have two choices: don't have sex or if you must, use birth control.

For most of you, being sexually active is far in the future. But when and if you do decide to become sexually active (on your wedding night or before), you should know the different methods of birth control that are available. You'll notice that not one of them can absolutely guarantee that you won't get pregnant.

The next three pages describe the most common birth control methods available, including how they work and how effective they are.

BIRTH CONTROL CHART

Condom

Also known as a "rubber," a condom is like a tight-fitting balloon that fits over a man's penis and collects the semen when the man ejaculates. Like the diaphragm and sponge, a condom is a *barrier method* of contraception. It works by keeping the sperm from reaching the egg by physically blocking their passage into the vagina.

If a man uses it correctly along with a spermicide or contraceptive foam, a condom is about 98 percent effective in preventing pregnancy. Besides abstinence, it is also the best protection against AIDS and other sexually transmitted diseases (STDs).

You may ask, *Why aren't condoms 100 percent effective?* In rare cases a condom can burst or tear, or it may have a defect to begin with, such as a small hole. Thus, the semen (and germs) can leak out of the condom and pass into the woman's vagina. The condom may also slip off during withdrawal of the penis.

Diaphragm

A diaphragm is a small rubber cup that fits over the cervix and blocks the sperm from going into the uterus and fallopian tubes. It's used with contraceptive cream or jelly that kills sperm.

If used carefully (and after some practice), a diaphragm is 97 percent effective. It must stay in place six to eight hours after sex.

A diaphragm is not effective if it's inserted improperly (not placed over the cervix) or if it's not used with spermicide. It must be inserted no more than six hours before sex.

Birth Control Pill

Called simply "the pill," it is made out of artificial hormones that stop ovulation from occurring by suppressing FSH and LH production. Birth control pills must be prescribed by a doctor and taken every day.

If used correctly, they are 99 percent effective. The most common failure of the birth control pill is not taking it correctly.

Although the pill is considered safe for most teens, there are some relative risks that should be discussed with your doctor.

Norplant

Containing similar hormones that the pill does, Norplant is a device consisting of several small capsules containing a long-acting progestin hormone. The device is implanted under the skin, and a constant low dose of progestin is released.

It's 98 to 99 percent effective, and depending on the type, it lasts from three to five years.

IUD

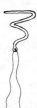

The IUD, which stands for intrauterine device, is a small copper device that is put inside the uterus during minor surgery. It keeps the fertilized egg from implanting and growing in the uterus.

It's 95 to 98 percent effective. However, the IUD can put a young woman at risk for severe pelvic infections, which will make it hard for her to get pregnant later on.

Generally, IUDs are not recommended for teens because of their high complication rate.

Vaginal Spermicides

These suppositories, creams, and jellies kill sperm. They are put up into the vagina before intercourse.

When used alone (and correctly), they're 80 to 95 percent effective. If used with a condom or diaphragm, they are 99 percent effective. They also offer some protection against STDs.

Sponge

Similar to the diaphragm, this small, soft, cup-shaped sponge is made of polyurethane. It is put inside the vagina and fits over the cervix. It contains chemicals that kill sperm. Since it also absorbs sperm, it acts as a barrier as well. Unlike a condom, you don't have to put in a new one for each sex act. Each sponge lasts 24 hours and should be kept in for 24 hours after sex.

If used carefully, it's 92 to 95 percent effective. As a barrier method of contraception, it also decreases the risk of STDs. On the down side, cases of TSS have been linked with use of the sponge, and unpleasant vaginal odor can be a problem.

"Natural" or Rhythm Method

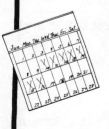

A woman charts the times when she ovulates (and therefore is most likely to get pregnant), and then makes sure she doesn't have sex during those times. This may involve several "fertility awareness" techniques, including charting monthly cycles, following basal body (vaginal) temperatures, and following cervical mucus changes.

If done correctly, this method is 80 to 98 percent effective. The trick is knowing precisely when ovulation occurs—not an easy thing to know, especially when ovulation times may vary. The fertility awareness techniques mentioned above are designed to assist a woman in "reading" her body from month to month.

Well, My Friend Said That . . .

There are some pretty wild stories floating around out there about sex. Most of them are wrong. How many of these myths have you accepted as "The Truth"?

Myth #1*: If you jump up and down after having sex, you can't get pregnant because the sperm will fall out.*

The Truth: Sperm travel fast. They're in the cervix within seconds, no matter how much jumping you do!

Myth #2*: You can't get pregnant the first time you have sex.*

The Truth: Ten percent of all teen pregnancies occur in the first month girls begin having sex. Fifty percent occur in the first six months!

Myth #3*: If you don't go "all the way," you can't get pregnant.*

The Truth: If sperm is released even near, not necessarily in, the vagina, they may still swim to the uterus and fertilize the egg.

Myth #4*: If a guy withdraws (pulls out his penis before ejaculating), you can't get pregnant.*

The Truth: A small amount of semen is released before a guy ejaculates. So even if a guy withdraws his penis, you can still get pregnant.

Myth #5*: You can't get pregnant during your period.*

The Truth: Although rare, you *can* have a short cycle and ovulate right on the heels of your last period.

Safe Sex

You've probably heard a lot about safe sex, but what does it really mean?

Lately the meaning has changed. "Safe" used to mainly mean safe as in "preventing pregnancy." Today, it means not only avoiding an unwanted pregnancy, but avoiding sexually transmitted diseases (such as AIDS) as well.

Actually, the term *safe sex* is misleading. You can never be completely safe from either pregnancy or disease when you have sex.

Check out the chart on birth control on pages 75–77 to find out which methods are safest for not getting pregnant. The safest method for preventing disease is use of condoms.

Sexually Transmitted Diseases

You've also probably heard about sexually transmitted diseases (STDs), but you may not realize how deadly they can be.

For example, AIDS is an STD. Right now, there is no cure for AIDS, and most everyone who has developed AIDS so far has eventually died from it.

You also may not be sure how you get STDs.

You get them by having sex with someone who has or carries one of the STDs. A man who's infected passes an STD to a woman through his semen or other body fluids.

Right now, STDs are a big problem. A lot of people have them. Unfortunately, a lot of those people are young. Nearly one-third of the people with STDs are teens.

Here's a quick rundown of common STDs:

AIDS. AIDS stands for **a**cquired **i**mmune **d**eficiency **s**yndrome. At present, there is no cure for AIDS, but there is hope. Effective treatments are being developed and used, and as you read this, the research continues for newer treatments, a vaccine, and even a cure.

AIDS is caused by a virus called HIV (**h**uman **i**mmunodeficiency **v**irus). HIV severely limits a person's ability to fight off infections. An AIDS patient, therefore, is prone to catching all sorts of deadly diseases, like certain forms of tuberculosis and cancer.

AIDS is spread through sexual intercourse. It can also be spread by:

- Sharing needles conta- minated by the AIDS virus. (This generally occurs among drug users. When you go to your doctor's office or to the hospital, any needle used on you is brand-new and sterile. A new needle is used on every person, so don't worry!)

WATCH OUT!

Only latex condoms, not membrane condoms, protect against the hepatitis B virus, Cytomegalovirus, and AIDS virus. Of course, if a condom tears or leaks, it offers no protection.

- Receiving a transfusion of contaminated blood or blood products. (Blood is now tested for HIV in the United States. However, testing didn't begin until 1985, so people who received transfusions before then were at risk of contracting the virus. Some of these people now have AIDS.)

- Passed from a pregnant woman to her unborn child or to a newborn baby during breast-feeding.

A lot still isn't known about AIDS. Experts agree that it is passed from an infected person to an uninfected one through body fluids.

They do know, however, that HIV can't be contracted through casual contact. You can't "catch it" by hugging, touching, or breathing the same air as an AIDS patient.

Researchers are continuing to make advances in their search for a cure for AIDS. Hopefully, there will be a cure within the next decade.

Genital Herpes. This is a virus that causes painful blisters or open sores anywhere on the genitalia or sometimes in or around the mouth. While the blisters last a few weeks, then go away, the herpes virus does not. It stays in your system, and the blisters may come back. While the blisters are present, you are very contagious.

Herpes can be treated with prescription drugs to shorten the duration and severity of the symptoms. However, it cannot be cured.

Genital Warts. These are caused by a virus related to the one that causes common warts. Genital warts are hard, painless, warty-looking lesions that appear on the sex organs or around the anus.

Doctors either prescribe a cream or lotion drug to get rid of them, or they may freeze them off or laser them. If the warts are large enough, they may have to be surgically removed. Even after they are treated, they may come back.

Chlamydial Infections. These are the most common type of STD. However, chlamydial infections often do not show any symptoms,

---

DO YOU KNOW WHAT'S REALLY SCARY ABOUT STDs?

- Anyone who has sex is at risk.

- Sometimes the symptoms don't show up for months (if ever). You can't even tell you're sick, so you don't get treatment. If this is the case, you may spread the disease.

- You can get more than one STD at the same time from one person.

- STDs affect the health of women more severely than men. They can make a woman infertile and have been linked to cervical cancer.

- They can kill you.

so people with the disease may pass it on to others without even knowing it!

Once the disease progresses, women may feel itching or burning in the genital area, as well as have a vaginal discharge. Men may find it painful to urinate and have a watery discharge come out of their penis.

Chlamydia can be treated by antibiotics. If left untreated, however, chlamydia can lead to a disease called PID (**p**elvic **i**nflammatory **d**isease) and sterility in women and boys.

Gonorrhea ("the clap"). Unfortunately, more teens than ever are suffering from gonorrhea. In fact, in recent years, girls ages 15 to 19 have caught it at a rate that's greater than for any other age group.

Like chlamydia, gonorrhea often doesn't show any symptoms. If symptoms do appear, a woman may experience a thick, creamy vaginal discharge, feel pain while urinating, and have some bleeding from her cervix. The disease can also sometimes invade the whole body, causing rashes, arthritis, and heart and central nervous system infections. If left untreated, it can cause PID and sterility.

Gonorrhea can be treated with antibiotics.

Syphilis. People with syphilis develop painless sores on their genitalia or mouth. Syphilis can be treated with antibiotics. If left untreated, this disease can lead to heart disease, brain damage, blindness, and even death.

Trichomoniasis. This is a common cause of vaginitis (irritation or inflammation of the vagina). Women with this disease usually suffer from vaginal itching, pain while urinating, and a smelly, frothy, greenish brownish discharge. This disease can be treated with antibiotics.

Hands Off, Please!

We don't need to tell you that kids your age are growing up fast. But no guy should ever push you into anything you're not ready for, even if it's just a hug or holding hands!

If a guy ever makes you feel uncomfortable, don't be afraid to tell him so. And if he touches you in ways you don't want to be touched, tell him to stop. After all, if he was pawing away at a friend, wouldn't you try to help her? You wouldn't do anything less for yourself, would you?

We know that it's hard to say no. You worry that the guy won't like you, or the other kids might think you're uncool. But, in the end, saying yes won't make anyone like you. People will end up not respecting you. Even worse, you probably won't like yourself!

CHAPTER 7

Roller-Coaster Emotions

"Until this year, her life had flowed along with rhythmic evenness. Now all that was changed. She was filled with a discontent, an anger about herself, her life, her family, that made her think she would never be content again."

—Sara Godfrey in Betsy Byars's *The Summer of the Swans*

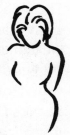

At this time in your life, not only is your body changing, everything is changing—your feelings toward boys, your best pals, and your parents.

Your feelings especially toward yourself are also changing. For instance, friends who you enjoyed spending every minute with last year, now seem boring. Sometimes you may get super-excited about the changes you're going through, then a minute later, you may feel down in the dumps about your new responsibilities and pressures.

It's a wild ride—but it's one that every girl takes. It's all part of growing up and into yourself.

Boys, Boys, Boys!

It used to be that boys were only good for teasing and for hitting baseballs with. Now, suddenly, guys you thought of as only buddies are looking pretty darn hunky. And there's a whole new world of feelings and experiences to get used to!

RELATIONSHIPS

Even though at times you may feel like a grown-up—especially with a new grown-up body—chances are you're not emotionally ready for a heavy-duty relationship. So, be patient. There's no need to rush into any relationship, even if you and a guy really like each other. Remember, you've got your whole life to meet and date boys!

Besides, at your age, your attention wanders every which way. Hold back on getting too involved in a relationship, because next week, you just might have your eye on an entirely new guy, and you may wish you had never gotten so serious!

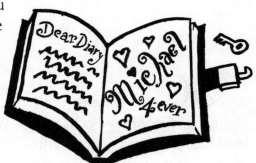

CRUSHES

You may be in the midst of your first crush—on the 17-year-old tennis coach at your club or maybe even Tom Cruise (you've seen all of his movies 13 times—a school record!). Whomever you've got your sights on, all you know is that you find yourself hopelessly daydreaming about him for hours!

While crushes may at times feel overwhelming, they're part of the process of discovering boys.

Sure, you may sometimes have a crush on the strangest people—your church minister, the bus driver, or the mailman—but in general, crushes are pretty harmless. However, keep in mind that crushes are usually a one-way ride to romance. Chances are, the guy you've got a crush on will never become more than just a crush. For example, no matter how charming, pretty, and talented you are, it's a long shot that you and Christian Slater will ever start dating!

So be careful not to let daydreaming substitute for real life. And every once in a while, stop drooling over your life-sized poster of your fave star and get out and meet some real-life guys!

TONGUE-TIED

During puberty, it's also not uncommon to find yourself suddenly shy around guys. It used to be you could talk for hours with a boy without even noticing how blue his eyes were or how cute that little dimple in his cheek was. Now that your romance eyes have opened, you may also be noticing that you can barely mumble a hello to a boy, let alone an entire sentence.

What do you do when you find yourself becoming speechless around guys? For starters, remember that even though they're members of the opposite sex, they're humans first, boys second! By thinking of them as *people,* not boys with a capital B, you may cut down on some of your anxiety.

Also keep in mind that any guy you talk to is probably just as nervous as you are. After all, he's entering puberty, too, and experiencing many of the same feelings as you are.

When you know you're going to be one-on-one with a guy, it's a good idea to come prepared with a few pre-planned topics, such as a paper you both have been assigned in

English class or the latest movies you've seen. By having a few safe topics of conversation up your sleeve, you'll never be left with nothing to talk about.

FLIRTY FRIENDS

Remember, too, that right about now your girlfriends are also going gaga over guys—and that will take some getting used to. One minute you have a perfectly normal best pal with whom you can talk about everything from school to parent problems. Now, suddenly, she's got only one subject on the brain: boys.

If you find yourself in this sticky situation, talk to your friend. Tell her that while you don't mind a bit of boytalk, you wish she would talk about a few other topics as well. Your friend will probably realize that she's become a boy bore and snap out of it.

Of course, there's always the chance that in a few weeks you'll become just as boy crazy as your friend. Then the two of you can gab about guys for hours!

Cliques

"I'm confused. Sometimes girls act nice, and then they are mean. There's this group. There's that group. Some ignore you. Some talk to you."

—Nichole Kennedy, age 12, Loveland, Colorado

Once you pass the age of 9 or 10, a funny thing happens. Girls start traveling around in packs. Girls who used to be perfectly capable of walking on their own now seem to be able to take steps only when surrounded by their best buddies. Not only that, but everyone has to dress the same way, wear their hair the same way, and talk the same way. It's as if, overnight, your pals turn into a pack of identical Barbie dolls! And suddenly, the school's filled with tight cliques. Sometimes you may feel like the only person on the outside.

Why do girls form "crowds"? A lot of times, the girls may feel insecure. Just like you, they're not sure who they are right now. They're feeling shaky about their changing bodies, their new feelings toward guys, and where they fit in the new social scheme. So, to make themselves feel better, they surround themselves with friends who look and act just like them.

What should you do if you don't seem to fit into a clique? Continue to be yourself—which means smiling and talking to the people you like and the people who like you. Try to stay open to new people and opportunities, and soon you'll find yourself with some fast friends.

It might also help to become active in a club or a sport where you're likely to be included in a circle of friends who share common interests.

What if you're in a clique that seems suffocating? The key thing to do is to be yourself, regardless of what any of your pals think or say. If you're buddies with kids whom your clique deems "nerdy," don't drop them. If you're into needlepoint, which your clique labels completely "uncool," don't drop the hobby. Only by staying true to yourself will you feel good about yourself, no matter what the clique says.

You'll also discover that, in the end, it's the only way to gain respect. Your true friends will stand behind you. And the ones who don't weren't really true friends to begin with.

Remember that peer pressure can be a powerful force. And, as you get older, it only gets worse as the stakes get higher (like when a certain crowd wants you to drink or do drugs). By setting your boundaries now, you can start building the self-esteem that will get you through any high-pressure situations later.

Fading Friendships

Around this time, you might find yourself growing apart from your very best pals. A girlfriend you've confided in since kindergarten may find a new best friend. Or one day you may realize you have nothing to talk about with her anymore.

As you and your friends try to figure out who you are, it's normal to find yourself attracted to new friends. Sometimes you and an old friend will eventually become great pals again. But, even if that doesn't happen, you'll both find new friends to take each other's place. And always try to part on friendly terms.

Parent Problems

"My dad told me the other day that I keep disobeying him and my mom. I guess it's true. They tell me not to do it, and I do it!"

—Gia Lewis, age 10, Thousand Oaks, California

If you're like many preteens, you and your parents have had a pretty harmonious relationship until now. Sure, you've had your fair share of fights—like the time you threw a fit because Dad wouldn't let you adopt the dozen homeless kittens someone had dumped at the supermarket. But now, ever since you hit puberty, your home has become a battlefield! You may find you and your mom tussling over such issues as how late you can stay out, who you can go out with, and how much makeup you can wear. Name the topic, and you're probably fighting over it.

What's Going On?

Your interactions with your parents are a normal part of growing up. You're beginning the slow process of creating a separate space from them.

In This Corner . . . You!

When you were a child, your parents were the most important people in your life. You wanted to spend all of your time with them. In your eyes, they were pretty perfect.

Now that you're older, you want more independence. Sometimes you'd rather go shopping alone than with the family clan. Plus you're testing your new grown-up status to see how far you can push it with your parents.

Friends are also becoming more important in your life. While you used to look forward to those Saturday afternoon family hikes, now those hikes are looking a little tame. You'd rather hang out with your girlfriends listening to the latest rap songs and doing your nails.

While it's normal to sometimes prefer to spend time with your friends instead of your parents, all of these changes are naturally going to cause some tension at home.

And in This Corner . . . Mom and Dad!

From your parents' point of view, you're growing up—and fast. Naturally, they have mixed feelings about it.

While your parents may be pleased to see you growing into a young woman, they also can't quite adjust to the fact that you aren't their baby anymore. They see you moving into the world of boys, dating, and makeup, and they miss the little girl you used to be. They're also scared that you might get hurt out in what they view as the big, bad world. So they hold on to you even more tightly.

And the Winner Is . . . Both of You!

During this time of transition, keep the lines of communication open with Mom and Dad. Let them know how *you're* feeling, and ask them how *they're* feeling. And don't forget to tell them you love them. After all, you do!

Be careful also not to push any newfound freedoms too far. For example, if your parents extend your Saturday night curfew from 8 o'clock to 9 o'clock, be smart and arrive home at the stroke of 9. If they agree that you can wear lipstick to school, don't sneak on blush and mascara as well.

Play by the rules and you'll cut down on any fighting and gain your parents' respect. Only by showing them that you can handle new responsibilities will they give them to you—without a big blowout!

With time, as you and your family adjust to the changes, tensions will lessen. Soon, these turbulent times will be a distant memory. You'll look back and wonder how you ever spent so much time arguing over so many silly things!

One Day You're Up, the Next You're Down

"I've been really sensitive lately. I cry a lot over silly things. One day my brother will say something and I won't get mad; the next day he'll say something and I get mad and want to cry. I'm just super moody."
—Meredith Chinn, age 9½, Newport Beach, California

Puberty often brings those crazy-making "mood swings" you've probably heard about. One minute you feel like you're ready to be the first female president. The next, you're so depressed you can barely get out of bed.

Part of your moodiness comes simply from being in transition. You're not a child anymore, but you're not an adult either. You may not even be a teen yet! That's a hard place to be in. One day you may hate your dad because he treated you like a baby and wouldn't let you stay up until 10 o'clock for a special TV show. The next, you're mad at your parents because they expected you to dress up and act all grown-up at one of their silly parties.

Puberty is a time of great expectations and great disappointments. You may wait excitedly for a big dance at school, then be crushed when the guy you like doesn't ask you to dance. You may have been looking forward to your 12th birthday bash with all your best pals for months. But the day it arrives, you feel like being alone and wish everyone would just go home.

You may take out your frustration on others or even on yourself. You may beat yourself up with thoughts like *you're no good, you're not nice enough,* or *how could anyone like you?*

How can you cope with all these overwhelming emotions? For starters, get them out. Write down your feelings in a journal or a song, or talk them out with a trusted adult or a friend.

Believe it or not, it also helps to get regular exercise. Working out is a super way to work out frustrations—even if you have only 10 minutes to spend dancing to your favorite song.

Also, block out some private time each day. Let this time be just for yourself—time to do whatever you want, even if it's just hanging out with your cat.

The key to getting through any rough emotional moments is to accept yourself. Accept the fact that sometimes you'll be up, sometimes down. Sometimes you'll feel lonely and think that no one understands you. Sometimes you may not want to do the things you always used to like to do.

It's okay to be uncertain and confused. Ask any one of your friends. If they're honest, they'll tell you that they're feeling the exact same way you are!

But remember that this time of roller-coaster emotions won't last forever. As you continue to grow up and learn about yourself, the moodiness will most likely go away. You'll feel more confident about yourself, who you are, and where you fit in.

CHAPTER 8

Candy for Breakfast, Chips for Lunch: Eating Right

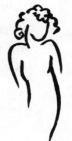

"I have a basic idea of the four food groups. Sometimes I don't always get enough fruit and vegetables I need in a day. But I also work out usually. So I'd say I'm in better shape than a lot of kids at my school."

—Jennifer Jones, age 13, Billings, Montana

Now that your body's growing and developing at a dramatic rate, it's more important than ever that you eat right. As you approach your teens, you have special nutritional requirements. You need extra energy to keep up with all of those preteen activities, like school dances and sports.

New studies also show that the better you eat now, the less likely you are to run into such health problems as heart disease when you're an adult.

While an occasional nibble-out on something wicked—barbecued potato chips or ultra-fudge brownies with extra walnuts—won't hurt, you'll feel better and be healthier if you stick to a healthy diet.

The Fab Four

Foods are broken down into four different groups. The best diets are those that choose from all four groups. Only by eating a varied, well-balanced diet can your body get all the nutrients it needs. With a varied diet, it's also less likely you'll burn out on the healthy stuff. If you ate the same exact foods each day, even hot fudge sundaes would start getting boring!

The four food groups are:

- **Milk products,** such as cheese, cottage cheese, yogurt, and milk. Dairy products are good sources of calcium, which helps to strengthen bones and teeth.

- **Fruits and vegetables.** These are a good source of vitamin C, which is found in fruits such as oranges and grapefruits and in vegetables such as tomatoes and broccoli. Vitamin C is important in maintaining the connective tissue in our bodies.

  Fruits and vegetables also contain potassium, which helps the kidneys as well as the heart and other muscles to function properly. The fiber in fruits and veggies also helps you to digest food.

- **Grains,** such as cereals, bread, rice, and pasta. These foods are a major source of complex carbohydrates, which supply readily available energy to the body in the form of blood sugar. They also contain essential vitamins and fiber. In addition, whole grains supply iron, which is very important for growing girls.

- **Meat or meat substitutes,** such as poultry, fish, shellfish, eggs, nuts, peanut butter, legumes (dried peas and beans), and tofu. These foods are rich in protein. Protein is needed to help build up your cells and body tissues. It also helps your body digest food and form hormones, among other important functions.

Daily Diet

Each day, try to eat the following foods:

- Three to five servings of vegetables. One serving equals ½ cup.

- Two to four servings of fruit. One medium piece of fruit, such as an apple or an orange or ½ cup of fruit juice equals one serving.

- Seven to eleven servings of grain products. One serving equals one slice of bread, one ounce of cereal, or ½ cup of pasta or rice.

- Three to four servings of milk products. One serving equals a cup of lowfat milk or yogurt.

- Three to four servings of meat or meat substitutes. One to two ounces from this food group equals one serving.

- Fats (including butter, oil, mayonnaise, and salad dressing) and sweets in limited quantities will make up the rest of your needed calories.

Food Pyramid

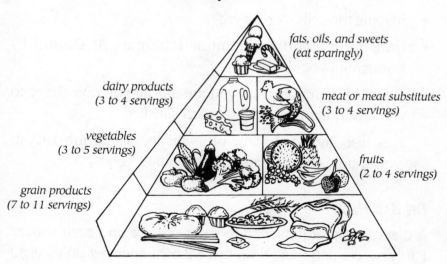

fats, oils, and sweets
(eat sparingly)

dairy products
(3 to 4 servings)

meat or meat substitutes
(3 to 4 servings)

vegetables
(3 to 5 servings)

fruits
(2 to 4 servings)

grain products
(7 to 11 servings)

Facts on Fat

"Jack Sprat could eat no fat, his wife could eat no lean,
And so betwixt the two of them, they licked the platter clean."
—Mother Goose rhyme

Do you ever feel like Jack Sprat? Feeling like if you dare eat anything with fat in it, you'll blow up like a balloon? Or maybe you feel like Jack's wife, eating fat all the time. Neither of these nursery rhyme characters has it right. One of the keys to good health is *eating fats in moderation*.

THE GOOD NEWS

You may be wondering why you should include any fat in your daily diet. After all, you hear a lot about the importance of lowfat diets.

While you don't want to overdose on fat, not eating enough can be dangerous. Fats perform many important functions in your body, such as:

- helping your brain develop
- helping to build cells
- helping the cells store energy
- transporting certain vitamins (vitamins A, D, and E) throughout your body
- signaling your body that you are full, so you don't have to eat large quantities of food to feel satisfied

Fats also give food some of its tastiness. But this isn't to say you should eat your heart out on fats!

THE BAD NEWS

A diet high in fat may lead to heart disease and even cancer. Fats also contain more than twice the calories per unit weight as carbohydrates or protein. Ounce for ounce, they can cause more unwanted weight gain than other foods, which can ultimately lead to high blood pressure, diabetes, and other health problems. So, what's the key to eating fat and maintaining good health? Eat fats *only in moderation.*

SATURATED VS. UNSATURATED FATS

The two kinds of fat you hear a lot about are saturated and unsaturated fats. What's the difference? Saturated fats are found mostly in products such as lard, meats, egg yolks, and dairy products. They're also found in some plant foods, such as coconut oil.

Unsaturated fats are found mostly in plant oils, such as corn and olive oil. They provide fats that are essential to our bodies that our bodies can't produce themselves, and in general they are thought to be healthier for our bodies than saturated fats.

FINDING FATS

You may be eating foods that have a heavy fat content without even knowing it. For example, muffins, hot dogs, and many types of crackers are loaded with fat.

What other foods have a high fat content?

- fried foods (french fries, fried chicken, doughnuts)
- rich foods (pastries, ice cream, heavy sauces)
- greasy foods (bacon)
- toppings (butter, margarine, mayonnaise)

If you find your diet is too heavy on fats, cut down by using these fat-trimming tips:

- Avoid rich sauces and gravies.

- Eat baked, broiled, steamed, poached, or grilled meats instead of fried foods.

- When seasoning meat or vegetables, substitute herbs and spices for butter or margarine.

- Drink lowfat milk instead of whole milk.

- Instead of eating french fries, try a baked potato, which has no fat.

- Use plain lowfat yogurt in place of sour cream.

CARBOS: THE GOOD AND THE BAD

Don't let the term *carbohydrates* confuse you. There are actually two types of carbos, complex and simple. Complex carbohydrates are found in whole-wheat breads, cereals, beans, pasta, and even fruits and veggies. These complex carbos should make up 50 to 60 percent of your diet each day.

Simple carbohydrates, on the other hand, refer to mostly pure sugar—high in calories with little nutritional benefit. Candy, sodas, sugary breakfast cereals, doughnuts, and fruit juices are loaded with simple carbohydrates. It's okay to nibble once in a while on these simple carbo foods, but to keep your body growing and running smoothly, load up on the complex carbos!

Drink Your Milk!

During puberty, your body needs more calcium than during any other time in your life. Your growing bones need the added calcium to grow into their full potential and to ensure that the amount of new bone you produce now is enough to last you a lifetime.

As women grow older they're prone to *osteoporosis,* a loss of bone volume. You can help prevent this disease now by getting your bones off to a healthy start.

As long as you're adding dairy products to your daily diet, you should have no problem getting enough calcium. Other foods rich in calcium include broccoli, greens (such as spinach and kale), and almonds.

If, however, you eat little or no dairy products, you may need calcium supplements. Ask your doctor for more information.

Become an Iron Woman

As you approach your teens, you also need more iron than ever before. In fact, many girls and boys suffer from a disease called *iron-deficiency anemia,* caused by a lack of iron. Anemia can make you tired and listless.

It's also possible to lose iron during your menstrual period.

Foods rich in iron include:

- strawberries
- apple, prune, or tomato juice
- broccoli
- green peas
- sweet potatoes
- spinach
- bran flakes with raisins
- oatmeal, Cream of Wheat
- pork, beef, or veal
- molasses
- navy, lima, and lentil beans

If you suspect you're not getting enough iron in your diet or if you're into a strenuous workout program, see your doctor about the possibility of needing iron supplements.

Iron deficiency in female athletes may occur due to a combination of several things: inadequate intake (as these girls tend to diet more), menstrual loss, and increased needs due to expansion of lean body tissue and blood volume throughout training. The more tissue and blood a girl has, the more iron she needs to take care of these tissues.

TAKE YOUR VITAMINS

Your mom may remind you to take your vitamins, but are they really necessary?

Vitamins are compounds needed in tiny quantities to keep the body's cells functioning properly. In general, if you're eating a well-balanced diet, you shouldn't need to take vitamin supplements.

In fact, too many vitamins can be too much of a good thing. Excessive vitamin A can cause peeling of the skin, increased pressure on the brain, changes in bones, and hair loss. Too much vitamin D can lead to a calcium buildup in the blood, which could lead to kidney stones. Taking too much vitamin C may also lead to kidney stones. Excessive vitamin E can interfere with the metabolism of other vitamins, cause bleeding problems, or cause an upset stomach.

The Not-So-Fab Four

Now that you know what foods to eat, here are some food products to avoid. The big baddies are:

Cholesterol

Cholesterol is a waxy, fatty substance found only in animal products such as meat, egg yolks, and cheese. There's good evidence that eating too much cholesterol can ultimately lead to heart disease and heart attacks.

In addition, some families have a genetic or inherited tendency for high cholesterol. Make sure you tell your doctor about your family's medical history so she or he can advise you.

Sugar

Sugar is often disguised in the food you eat. Maple syrup, ketchup, jam, fruit juices, soft drinks, and breakfast cereals are often loaded with sugar.

Eating too much sugar can give you cavities and cause unwanted weight gain. While sugar gives your body a quick boost, after the initial effect wears off, it leaves you more tired than before.

Salt

If you're like most people, salting your food is second nature. But next time, halt before you salt. One teaspoon of salt contains 2,800 milligrams of sodium. Your body needs only a fraction of that amount to meet its daily sodium requirements.

Excessive salt intake can lead to high blood pressure and other related health problems. It can also cause you to retain water and become bloated.

While foods high in salt are often hard to avoid (especially when someone passes you the guacamole and chips!), try to

> **JUNK FOOD JUNKIES**
>
> If you're struck by a snack attack and can't resist diving into the cookie jar, take heart. As long as you eat healthful foods throughout the day, you can indulge in a handful of cookies from time to time.
>
> Keep in mind, however, that junk foods are filled with calories, fat, and salt, and are short on essential vitamins and nutrients. So the key isn't giving up your favorite junk food, but eating it in moderation.

pass on highly salted foods whenever possible. Also avoid any fast foods or highly processed luncheon meats, which are usually laden with sodium.

Caffeine

Even if you're not a coffee drinker, you may be a big caffeine consumer. Tea, soft drinks, and chocolate all contain large doses of caffeine.

Why is it best to avoid caffeine? Because large amounts can cause many side effects, among them anxiety, stomachaches, sleeplessness, and irritability. So the next time you reach for that diet Coke, grab a glass of water instead.

The Exercise Factor

Eating right is just half of the healthy body equation. The other half is making sure you get regular exercise.

With your busy schedule, you might wonder how you'd have enough time to exercise. Maybe the very word "exercise" makes you want to climb under your bed covers. Don't worry, though! Fitness doesn't have to be strenuous or time consuming. In fact, exercise can be a fun and exciting part of your day.

Why is exercise so important? First, it strengthens your heart and other components of your cardiovascular system. This is especially true of any exercise program that increases your breathing and heartbeat to your *target heart rate* (see page 107).

Second, exercise is a beauty prescription! It burns fat, tones muscles, and improves the appearance of skin and hair. It's also a mood and energy booster. All around, exercise is worth the time and trouble, since it makes you feel and look so good.

GETTING STARTED

You don't want to be sidelined with an injury, so you'll want to take some smart precautions before starting any new exercise program.

1. Talk to your family doctor. This is especially important if you've had any medical problems, are currently taking medication, or are recovering from an injury. Exercise is good for you, but not if it worsens a medical condition!

2. Suit up in proper workout clothes and shoes, essential for your comfort and safety. You'll feel best in well-fitted workout clothes made from absorbent material like cotton. You'll also want to wear an athletic bra, supportive halter top, or athletic swimsuit to support your breasts properly. Don't forget your feet, either! Athletic shoes especially made for your particular sport are helpful, but not essential.

> You can exercise, and even swim, during your period. In fact, workouts can reduce irritability, fatigue, and bloating related to menstruation. Some girls are more accident-prone during their periods because they have more difficulty concentrating. (Of course, it's always important to use caution during any physical activity.)

What is important are shoes that fit your feet, since too-snug or too-loose shoes create calluses or accidents.

3. Gently warm up your muscles and stretch before any vigorous activity. Always begin with a five-minute warm-up,

with slow movements that gradually increase your heart and breathing rate. Stretch your muscles like your pet cat does after a nap. Once you've warmed up, you're ready to go!

4. If you ever feel dizziness or sharp pain while exercising, stop. However, avoid suddenly stopping exercise once your heart has reached its target rate. Instead, slowly wind down your activities by walking until your heart returns to its normal rate.

5. Avoid dehydration by drinking plenty of water before, during, and after your workout. Some people carry a water sipper to refresh themselves while exercising. In hot climates, work out during the cooler morning or evening hours, or indoors, to avoid heatstroke. If you live in a climate with high humidity (80 percent or more), keep activity lower-paced to avoid straining the heart. Workouts in cold climates are safer and more comfortable when you dress in layers, and cover your mouth with an absorbent scarf that warms air as you breathe.

FAT-BURNING EXERCISE

Aerobic exercise refers to any activity where you reach your target heart rate and is one of the best ways to burn excess body fat. As a bonus, your brain produces a calming brain chemical called "serotonin," which makes you feel really good after an aerobic workout.

To maintain fitness, the body needs between thirty and sixty minutes of aerobic activities performed three to five days a week, according to the American College of Sports Medicine. To avoid boredom and to work all your muscle groups, it's best to vary your exercise routines. Here are some aerobic activities to give you ideas, and to show approximately how many calories they burn.

Activity	Approx. Calories Burned Per Hour*
Bicycling (5 mph)	190
Gymnastics	200
Racquetball	620
Roller Skating	275
Running	400
Skiing	460
Swimming	400
Tennis	330
Walking	230

*Based on female body weight of 110 pounds. Caloric rates will be slightly lower or higher for body weights lower or higher, respectively.

Finding Your Heart Rate

The target heart rate for girls ages 9 to 13 is between 135 and 155 beats per minute. The maximum average heart rate for your age group is 210 beats per minute. That means the fastest your heart can beat is 210 times in a minute. (To find your own specific maximum heart rate, subtract your age from 220. Your target heart rate is 65 to 75 percent of your maximum heart rate.)

It's a good idea to check your heart rate during exercise to make sure you are working out at your target heart rate. Never let it exceed your maximum heart heart. If your heart is beating too fast, slow down your activities. If your heart is below the target heart range, slightly increase your activities. To check your heart rate, put your thumb on your wrist or your throat. Count the number of times your heart beats during a ten-second period. Multiply that number by six to find your current per-minute heart rate.

TONING YOUR MUSCLES

Along with aerobic activity, some people do exercises that tone and tighten the muscles. Examples include sit-ups and crunches that tighten the abdominal muscles, or leg lifts to firm the gluteal (buttocks) region. Many young women use small barbells and stationary weightlifting equipment to tone their muscles. Female hormones prevent girls and women from developing bulky muscles, although you've probably seen female weight lifters whose restrictive diets exaggerate their muscle lines. Some female body builders take steroids to get larger muscles. Steroids contain testosterone, the hormone usually found only in males.

If you decide to use weights, you'll want to become informed about safety procedures. Consult a knowledgeable physical fitness teacher or trainer before attempting a weightlifting program.

The key to making exercise a regular part of your schedule is to finding a program you enjoy, whether it's bicycling, dancing, or tennis!

BEATING COUCH POTATO BLUES

"It's too hot!" "I'm too tired!" "Exercise is boring!" Some days, you'd rather take an S.A.T. exam than work out. Although it's okay to skip exercise occasionally (especially if you're ill), many people procrastinate or avoid exercise completely. Do you need help getting motivated to move your body? Try these tips below!

1. *The 15-minute trick:* Tell yourself, "I'm just going to exercise for 15 minutes. If at the end of 15 minutes, I feel like stopping, I will." Most of the time, once you've gone to the trouble of putting on your workout clothes and shoes, you'll keep going after 15 minutes.

2. After a workout: After a workout, indulge in your favorite activity like listening to music, going to the mall, or reading that new magazine. Pairing pleasure with exercise makes you more likely to enjoy it.

3. Get company: Solo exercising can sometimes feel lonely, so grab your best buddy and work out together.

4. Mix it up: The same old exercise, day in and day out, gets old after awhile. Vary your exercise routines to stir your interest and motivation.

5. Ink it in: You do lots of things that you'd rather not do (like homework and chores!). Would you ever go to school without brushing your hair or getting dressed? Of course not! Put exercise in the same non-optional category. Write a realistic exercise schedule you can live with—commit it to your calendar in ink!

HOOKED ON EXERCISE

Sometimes, people overdo their workouts in misguided attempts to lose weight faster or to avoid facing personal problems. Girls who overexercise risk permanent injury to their muscles and bones. Overexercising can lead to amenorrhea (when periods stop or are skipped), which leads to fragile bones in adulthood. Symptoms of exercise addiction include:

- Periods stop or skip months
- Irritability, low energy, burn-out
- Friends and family express concern over how much time is spent exercising
- Exercise interferes with schoolwork and friendships
- Refuses to stop exercising while ill or injured
- Unrealistic fears of sudden weight gain if she skips or reduces exercise

- If you or someone you know is overexercising, talk to your family doctor, school nurse, or counselor. Exercise addiction often masks emotional upsets such as grief, depression, and low self-esteem—issues needing the help of a treatment professional.

BODY FAT

More than ever today, "fat" has become an obscene word. But everyone's body carries some fat, and for health and beauty reasons, you wouldn't want it any other way. Some body fat is necessary for the body to operate, and to give the face and body a healthful, vibrant appearance. Extreme thinness is neither healthful nor attractive!

Before girls reach puberty, their bodies are normally 15 percent fat. At puberty, hormonal changes increase body fat to around 22 percent. Teenage Olympic gymnasts have about 14 percent body fat because of their rigorous training schedules.

You can measure your body fat with a painless electronic gauge that is taped or clipped to your hands. Many family physicians, weight loss counselors, and health food stores offer "fat testing" services. The cost is nominal and the procedure takes less than five minutes. Immersion in a water tank also measures body fat percentage. Some health clubs offer this type of service.

Some people's fat distributes in a way that looks like dimples, commonly called "cellulite." Cellulite is ordinary fat that many women develop below the buttocks. There are no exercises, diets, or creams that remove fat from selected locations. The best way to lose fat is through low-fat eating combined with regular aerobic exercise. Fat loss and gain occurs over the entire body. Water retention and loss—not fat—is responsible for changes in the appearance of breasts and face that some girls experience during weight changes.

Can I Trade in My Body for Niki Taylor's?

It can be hard in today's world to feel good about your body. You're bombarded with images of svelte, shapely models that fill the pages of fashion magazines and seem to populate every MTV video and every film. The message seems to be: If your body doesn't look perfect, something's wrong with you.

Nothing could be further from the truth!

First of all, bodies come in all shapes and sizes. There is no "perfect" body. A tall, thin body can be beautiful, but so can a short, curvy body. What makes a girl or woman beautiful is how she carries herself, not her dimensions!

You might feel better knowing that many of the models you see in fashion magazines don't look that way in real life. Many photos are airbrushed to rid them of any flaws. A model's thigh might be "trimmed" or her bust enhanced with shading. In the magazine ads for some movies, another woman's body is sometimes attached to the head of the actress!

While it's fun to flip through the pages of such magazines or zone out in front of MTV, don't get too hung up on the "perfect" bodies. There's much more to you than your body—like your terrific mind and personality, for starters!

Eating Disorders

"I have a friend. She's a model and she's really thin. She thinks she's fat, even though there's no meat on her stomach. I say, shut up! I worry that someday she could get anorexic."
—Jennifer Hirsch, age 13, Hillsborough, California

Except for cancer, eating disorders kill more girls than any other disease. Physicians classify eating disorders as a disease because they consist of addictive behaviors along with a diagnosis and a treatment program, or prognosis. Like other diseases, eating disorders are progressive conditions—meaning, the symptoms worsen when left untreated. If being deadly weren't enough, eating disorders also wreck a person's health and physical appearance.

Most girls who become eating disordered start innocently enough. They don't intend to kill or injure themselves! They just want to drop a few pounds, and then quickly lose control of their behavior. Instead of feeling thin, beautiful, and popular as they'd hoped, eating disordered girls suffer from fatigue, self-disgust, and depression.

According to the National Institute of Mental Health, almost five million Americans suffer from eating disorders—90 percent of them female. There are two types of eating disorders: anorexia nervosa and bulimia nervosa.

ANOREXIA NERVOSA

Anorexia nervosa is a deadly and debilitating eating disorder that causes people to starve themselves. The anorexic is often a young woman who believes her only sources of self-esteem come from being ultra-thin like a model or pop music star. When the scale registers a weight loss, she feels successful and in control. She ignores other people's comments that she's "too thin," believing others are jealous or trying to control her.

Dangers of Anorexia

Self-starvation is an addictive behavior that rapidly leads to health problems, including dehydration, malnutrition, electrolyte imbalances that can cause sudden death, heart conditions, and the development of excessive facial hair. Psychological problems associated with anorexia include depression, suicidal tendencies, feelings of worthlessness, and chronic fatigue.

People with anorexia have "distorted body images." This means that, although she is quite thin, she sees a fat person when looking at herself in the mirror. She never feels thin enough! In one study, anorexic girls estimated their bodies to be 74 percent larger than their actual size. Girls who participate in ballet and gymnastics are statistically more likely to engage in self-starvation out of pressures to achieve thinness.

Psychotherapy (often inpatient) is necessary to help the anorexic discover healthy ways to maintain her weight and self-esteem. Unfortunately, many anorexics resist getting help because of their fears of being controlled, criticism, or gaining weight. Every year, 2 to 8 percent of anorexic people die.

PATIENT PROFILE

Who is at risk for anorexia? Studies show that young females are more at risk than any other group. There are two peak at-risk times: between the ages of 12 and 14 and the ages of 17 and 18.

Most anorexics usually come from white, middle- to upper-class families. Their families typically place a lot of importance on achievement.

Often the patient is a so-called model child. Always willing to please, she gets good grades, usually bends to her parents' will, and stays out of trouble. Inside, however, she may feel that she has little control over her life.

In striving for approval and perfection, the anorexic turns to one thing she can "control" and make perfect: her body. She may start to diet to take off just those few extra pounds she feels make her body "flawed," but then she gets caught up in a potentially deadly diet.

Not content to lose 5 or even 10 pounds, she keeps on dieting, even if she loses much more weight than is healthy. During this process, she often denies feeling hungry or claims that just a few bites of food will fill her up.

Causes

After years of research, experts are still not sure what causes anorexia. While we've discussed some of the psychological factors leading to the disease, some experts believe that there also might be a physical component. Research is being done to determine if certain parts of the brain start to function improperly before and after the disease begins.

BULIMIA

You may also have heard of an eating disorder that is related to anorexia called *bulimia*. This is a condition in which people binge on large quantities of food, then purge by using laxatives or making themselves vomit.

After an eating binge, the bulimic person takes action to rid herself of the calories she's ingested. She purges the food by sticking her finger down her throat to induce vomiting, taking a laxative or amphetamine-like pill or drink, exercising excessively, or skipping meals for the rest of the day.

Unlike the emaciated thin body of the anorexic, most bulimics are overweight. Purging just can't rid the body of all the food ingested during a binge. Many girls who start with anorexia nervosa later switch to practicing bulimic behavior. It is rare for the reverse to occur.

Constant vomiting produces some scary side effects. Bulimics can suffer from low blood pressure and a high heart rate. Their faces and the whites of their eyes may become filled with broken blood vessels.

Further, their teeth may decay from having frequent contact with the acidic contents of the stomach. And their esophagus, the tube leading from the mouth to the stomach, can become inflamed or torn.

Dying to be Thin

Bulimia is lethal behavior! The most common cause of death among bulimics is suicide, both accidental (such as choking on one's own vomit) and deliberate. Purging and unbalanced diets play havoc with the body's electrolytes and other chemicals that regulate mood and energy levels. So, most bulimics feel depressed and tired—two feelings associated with suicidal behavior.

Some bulimics induce vomiting with syrup of Ipecac (commonly given to babies who ingest poison). This medicine has a cumulative effect that literally poisons and kills the person who uses it chronically. The most famous case of Ipecac poisoning related to an eating disorder happened when pop singer Karen Carpenter was found dead after repeatedly abusing the drug to lose weight.

OBESITY

People who are obese are severely overweight. It's caused by several things, among them overeating, heredity, or a nonactive lifestyle. Some people are prone to easy and quick weight gain, while other girls can eat a triple decker ice cream cone each night before bed and never gain an ounce.

Obesity can be tough psychologically. Many obese people feel alone and unaccepted. Physically, obesity takes its toll on a body and may ultimately cause high blood pressure, diabetes, or a stroke.

In the last decade, the number of obese American adults has increased by over 10 percent. The American Dietetic Association estimates that one in four U.S. children is obese—a whopping 54 percent increase compared with twenty years ago. Adolescent obesity is a growing concern among medical doctors at the National Center for Health Statistics, who worry these overweight teens will mature into sedentary, unhealthy adults. The main culprits blamed for the growing girth of Americans are high-fat diets and inadequate exercise.

Treatment for Eating Disorders

As doctors learn more about obesity, anorexia, and bulimia, they are discovering effective ways to treat these disorders. Treatment consists of a lot of psychological counseling for the patient and her family. Doctors will also map out a nutritional plan for the patient.

For the obese person, treatment consists of dietary counseling and planning with a nutritionist, an exercise program, and peer group counseling. There are now also many hospital- or clinic-based obesity programs for teens and their families.

For the anorexic, the main goal is to help her stabilize her body chemistry and gain weight. Often the patient has to be hospitalized for several weeks or months to get her body weight up.

It's essential that anyone suffering from an eating disorder gets as much support as possible from a caring medical staff and her family and friends. These disorders are devastating to go through, but with time and a lot of help, they can be overcome.

If you think that you may be suffering from an eating disorder—even from the early signs of the disease (you weigh yourself constantly, think about food all the time, or have drastically increased or decreased your food intake), don't hesitate to see a doctor. If seeing a doctor seems too scary, at least confide in a school counselor or a trusted adult. He or she can see that you get the help you need.

If you suspect that a friend is suffering from an eating disorder, don't keep it a secret. Your pal needs your help fast. Talk to your parents or another trusted adult about your friend. He or she can then take matters in hand and go about seeing that your friend gets help.

CHAPTER 9

*G*ood Sense News

> "I learned what drugs, smoking, and alcohol can do to you in a class at school. It really scared me. Especially the part about lung cancer.
>
> I learned a five-step way of saying no and staying out of trouble. I practice saying no with my mom."
>
> —Karen Cloutier, age 10, Albuquerque, New Mexico

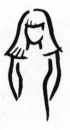

*F*rom your first kiss to driving your first car, you've got a lot of exciting "firsts" to look forward to. However, some "firsts" you're going to encounter in the next few years can do you a lot of harm, such as alcohol, drugs, and cigarettes. These substances are bad news, any way you look at them.

They can hurt your mind and body, get you in a lot of trouble, and even kill you. (Using them won't make you any more popular, either!)

Read on to find out exactly what makes these baddies so bad and why you should avoid them.

Want a Beer? No Thanks, I'll Pass!

Maybe you know a "hip" guy at school who brags about downing beer every weekend. Or a popular girl who sneaks wine coolers into her locker and shows them off at lunch.

While these kids may seem cool, what they're doing to their minds and bodies isn't cool at all.

SIDE EFFECTS

At first, alcohol gives a person an immediate buzz. It can cause a person to feel light-headed and have a temporary sense of well-being.

Some people get addicted to these feelings. In fact, it's all too easy to get hooked on alcohol. But the short-term buzz isn't worth the long-term damage.

Alcohol is called a "downer" because it slows down the body's central nervous system. That's why people who've had too much to drink slur their speech and stagger when they walk.

Alcohol alters moods and can cause normally cheerful people to become depressed. It also breaks down inhibitions. The more a person drinks, the more likely he or she will say something embarrassing or do silly things.

People who drink large amounts over a short period of time may become so drunk that they pass out, not even re-membering what happened to them. If their body can't handle all that liquor, they may have trouble breathing and even die.

Once the alcohol wears off, it's *still* no party. People some-times get what's called a hangover, which are bad side effects after the alcohol wears off. These can range from a headache and dizziness to nausea, fatigue, and irritability.

You don't have to drink to become a victim of alcohol. Every year lots of kids lose their lives due to alcohol-related car crashes, drownings, and other accidents.

Some people who drink suffer from a disease called *alcoholism*. This is when drinking becomes a way of life. Unable to stop, the alcoholic continues drinking even if he or she becomes out of control or passes out, or causes harm to others.

Alcoholics may start out as casual drinkers, then eventually find themselves putting alcohol before everything: family, friends, careers, even their own health.

Some families have a genetic tendency toward alcoholism. If you're from such a family, even one or two drinks can be harmful to you.

Chronic drinking is definitely deadly. It can lead to many serious problems, among them:

- damage to the brain, pancreas, and kidneys
- high blood pressure, heart attacks, and strokes
- inflammation and scarring of the liver, also known as cirrhosis
- stomach ulcers
- premature aging

Scary stuff, isn't it? You don't even have to think twice to figure out that alcohol is something to stay away from.

So the next time that cool guy at school brags about drinking beer, sip your seltzer water or juice with confidence!

Drugs? No Way, No How!

Just as you may know kids who drink, you probably know some who use drugs. Again, they make it sound like it's the super-hip thing to do.

But we're going to tell you the truth. Drugs—even pot—really can hurt you. They're very addicting, horrible for your body, and can even kill you. They also can cause emotional problems, leading you to withdraw from everyone you love, even yourself.

There are all sorts of drugs out there. Legal drugs are those that you can buy over the counter or through a prescription. But just because a drug is legal does not mean it isn't dangerous. Even aspirin, if taken in large amounts, can kill you.

Illegal drugs are those whose manufacture, sale, or purchase is against the law. Illegal drugs include marijuana, cocaine, and LSD.

MARIJUANA

A lot of kids use marijuana (also called pot), which is why you may hear that it's harmless. But that is not true.

Here are some of the side effects of this supposedly "harmless" drug:

- Chronic lung disease. In fact, because marijuana smokers try to hold smoke in their lungs for as long as possible, one marijuana cigarette can be as damaging to the lungs as four tobacco cigarettes.

- Temporary memory loss, loss of judgment, and sloweddown motor skills. New research shows that marijuana use can even result in permanent memory loss.

- Speeded-up heart rate and higher blood pressure.

- Bloodshot eyes.

- Dry mouth and throat.

- Increased appetite and thirst, which can lead to unwanted weight gain.

- Severe depression or anxiety.

- Panic attacks, which often strike first-time users.

Over the years, pot has gotten a lot more potent. You've no doubt heard people talking about using pot back in the 1960s for a "harmless" high. Because of better growing and breeding of the plant, the concentraton of THC (**t**etra**h**ydro**c**annabi-nol, the major mood-altering component of marijuana) is many times higher than it was in the 1960s. Marijuana is also sometimes mixed with other, more dangerous drugs.

Just as driving and drinking are a deadly duo, so are driving and smoking pot. Marijuana affects driving skills for at least four to six hours after smoking a single joint.

In addition, kids who use marijuana at an early age risk growing up to be losers. They lose ambition, can't make decisions or carry through with plans, have difficulty concentrating, and do poorly in school or at work. Many teens who wind up in drug treat-ment centers started using pot at an early age.

DESIGNER DRUGS

There's a new breed of drugs showing up at parties called "designer" drugs. These drugs, which are combinations of other drugs, are really dangerous because they're even more potent than the original drugs.

One designer drug you may have heard of is called "ecstasy." This drug causes a quick rush and disorienta-tion. It is very dangerous because it kills off brain cells. Once dead, brain cells do not regenerate or replace themselves.

COCAINE

Another drug you've probably heard about is cocaine, also called coke. A fine white powder, cocaine is usually inhaled through the nose. Even though coke is very expensive, more and more teens and other kids are trying it.

Cocaine makes a person feel "hyper" and extra-alert. It's a stimulant, which means it gives the body a giant jolt. It also gives a strong sense of euphoria or well-being, a sensation that the user tries to repeat over and over again. The heart rate speeds up. It can also cause the shakes, sweats, and restlessness. But as the drug wears off, the opposite effects occur. The user becomes depressed, anxious, or irritable and takes more cocaine to feel good again.

This is why cocaine is so addicting. Even one dose can cause the body to develop the uncontrollable need to have the drug again and again.

Because cocaine is expensive, some people throw away everything in pursuit of their cocaine habit. It can cause teens to start stealing, or even push them into prostitution in a desperate attempt to make enough money to buy more coke.

Cocaine causes many harmful side effects, including:

CHEAP AND DEADLY THRILLS

Some kids are getting high from inhaling common household substances, from nail polish remover to glue. While these substances may seem harmless, they've been responsible for many deaths.

Using inhalants, or "huffing," is becoming more popular. A recent study released by the National Institute on Drug Abuse in 1993 showed that one in every six eighth-graders had used some sort of inhalant in their life.

Why is huffing so deadly? The inhaled substances can cause breathing problems, destroy lung tissue, and damage kidneys. Users can black out or become panicky or depressed. Their hearts may also suddenly stop beating.

- dilated pupils, raised temperature, and high blood pressure
- hallucinations
- vomiting
- severe and chronic fatigue (the user is too wired to sleep)

- chronic coughing and nose bleeds
- sinus and upper respiratory tract congestion and damage

Ultimately, cocaine can cause seizures, heart failure, respiratory arrest, strokes, and possibly death.

CRACK

Crack is a rock form of cocaine that is usually smoked. Crack is a much more concentrated form of cocaine that rapidly reaches the brain and causes an immediate, intense high. Because of its immediate effects, crack is also highly addictive. Sometimes just one or two tries will get a person immediately hooked.

HOW TO TELL IF SOMEBODY IS USING DRUGS OR ALCOHOL

Be on the alert for these warning signs that a pal's getting caught up in the deadly cycle of alcohol and/or drug use.

Casual use: You start catching your friend telling little lies. She (or he) may disappear for periods of time with no explanation of where she's been.

Increased use: Your friend drops her after-school activities and hobbies. She starts pulling away from you and hanging out more with the "druggies." She's super-moody and may dress differently. She may even skip school.

Constant use: She drops you and other friends who don't use drugs. She's fighting with her parents, lying a lot, failing class, and skipping school often. She may even be stealing.

Serious addiction: She's lost weight and looks sickly. She may have a chronic cough if she's into pot or cocaine. She may not be able to remember things she should. She may also be paranoid or prone to fits of anger. She may drop out of school or get in trouble with the law.

LSD

LSD is another drug that was used a lot in the 1960s. Now it's popular again—and just as dangerous a drug as before.

Some of the "mild" effects of using LSD are mood swings and clouded judgment. But the scariest thing about LSD is that it causes hallucinations. Hallucinations are vivid images and thoughts that enter your mind as if you were dreaming— but you're awake. Sometimes these hallucinations are terrify- ing, like horrible nightmares. These "bad trips" can cause

OTHER DRUGS TO STAY AWAY FROM AND THEIR EFFECTS

"Speed" *a powerful stimulant*	nervousness, irritability, insomnia, nausea, hot flashes, sweating, heart palpitations, dryness of the mouth, confusion, severe anxiety, paranoia, death
"Downers" *depressants*	disorientation, slurred speech, sedation, seizures, coma, heart failure, and death
PCP *hallucino- genic drug*	distortion of reality and possible memory loss, lack of concentration, decreased blood pressure, breathing problems, feelings of super-human strength (which can cause a person to attempt dangerous stunts), coma, and death
Heroin *highly addictive narcotic*	drowsiness, delirium, loss of the sensation of pain, shallow breathing, nausea, panic attacks, insomnia, skin and blood infections, the risk of contracting AIDS or hepatitis through shared needles, coma, and death

extreme panic, leading people on LSD to jump out of a window, run into the middle of busy traffic, and do other life-endangering things *nobody* in their right mind would ever do! Moreover, recurring hallucinations—flashbacks—can suddenly seize a user long after the drug has worn off.

And What About Cigarettes? They'll Burn You, Too

When you were little, remember how gross it was to be around someone who smoked? The person probably continually coughed, smelled like an old ashtray, and had stained teeth and fingers.

Keep the image of that person in mind as you grow up and meet kids who will try to convince you to smoke. Tobacco is used by more kids (20 percent) than any other drug (yes, tobacco is considered a drug). Girls are particularly susceptible because many tobacco companies are targeting their ad campaigns toward women.

Perhaps the worst thing about smoking is that a few puffs now could make you hooked for life. With the exception of crack and cocaine, cigarette smoking is *the* most addictive habit known. In fact, 85 percent of adolescents who smoke two or more cigarettes a day will become regular smokers as adults. And breaking the habit is a long, hard process.

Smoking is a terrible thing to do to your body. You don't believe us? Take a look at the facts:

• An estimated 85 percent of cases of lung cancer in males and 75 percent in females are caused by cigarette smoking. What's worse, of the smokers who develop lung cancer, 87 percent eventually die from the disease.

- The risk of developing lung cancer increases with the number of years a person has been smoking, the number of cigarettes smoked per day, and the tar and nicotine content of the preferred brand of cigarettes.

- Even smoking cigarettes low in tar and nicotine puts smokers at risk for lung cancer.

- Smoking can also cause a host of other physical problems, such as respiratory disease (emphysema), heart disease, and mouth cancer. It can aggravate asthma and lead to lung infections.

Another reason not to smoke: concern for the health of others! Breathing "secondhand smoke" can cause problems. This sort of passive inhaling can result in respiratory disease and even death. In fact, according to the American Cancer Society's 1992 *Cancer Facts & Figures,* in the United States, approximately 53,000 people die annually as a result of breathing secondhand smoke.

CHAPTER 10

When You Have Medical Needs

"I'm pretty healthy and don't think about getting sick much. But one day last year I woke up feeling really awful. Turns out, I had strep throat. I was sick for about a week. But my mom gave me extra Popsicles and soup, which made me feel a lot better."

—Mary Lovell, age 12, Raleigh, North Carolina

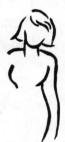

We've listed the most common problems that crop up during puberty and what you can do about them. Then all your fears about the gynecologist will be dispelled as you read a step-by-step account of what your first visit to the gynecologist will be like!

Vaginitis

Vaginitis, an inflammation or irritation of the vagina, is a very common problem. Sometimes bacteria are a direct cause, such as when bacteria in your stool get into your vaginal area from improper wiping (always remember to wipe yourself from front to back after going to the bathroom). Other times, certain conditions make your vaginal area more vulnerable to invasion by bacteria or other microorganisms—in particular, yeast (a.k.a. Candida)—that can cause vaginitis. Actually, this is quite common in females. For example, when you sit around in a wet bathing suit, wear underwear without a cotton crotch, or wear very tight jeans, the skin gets chafed and warm and moist—a condition these organisms love.

The vagina is very sensitive. Anything that alters its environment can cause vaginitis. Sometimes direct contact with a chemical irritant is also enough to make the area vulnerable to infection.

What are the symptoms? The most common one is vaginal discharge. This discharge is different from the clear or slightly yellow discharge you usually have. It may be smelly, irritating, or a color or consistency you've never seen before (and hope you never see again!).

Other symptoms include itching, as well as discomfort and burning when you urinate.

If you suspect you have vaginitis, see a doctor immediately.

COMMON CAUSES OF VAGINITIS

- soaps
- detergents
- bubble baths
- colored toilet paper
- sanitary napkins
- lubricants
- contraceptive foams or jellies
- rayon or nylon underwear
- douches/feminine hygiene sprays
- sand
- perfumes
- shaving creams
- antibiotics
- wet clothing
- tight clothes
- birth control pills

He or she will treat the infection by putting you on medication. The treatment could be a topical antifungal cream or vaginal suppository (where you insert a measured amount of medication into your vagina), or sometimes even an oral antibiotic.

AVOIDING VAGINAL INFECTIONS

- Avoid wearing tight clothes. If you're addicted to your skintight jeans, at least take them off a few hours each day!

- Wash your genital area well each day.

- Change your underwear each day. Also opt for cotton underwear instead of nylon, or at least underwear lined with a cotton crotch.

- Avoid sharing bathing suits or towels, even with your closest pals, as these can carry bacteria that cause infection.

- Change out of a wet bathing suit as quickly as possible.

- After going to the bathroom, wipe yourself from front to back. This will help avoid bringing any bacteria from your anal area to your vaginal opening.

- Don't douche or use feminine deodorant sprays.

- Avoid harsh soaps.

- Change your sanitary napkins frequently.

Bladder Infection

Also known as a urinary tract infection, a bladder infection is caused by bacteria in the bladder. Girls and women are more at risk than boys and men for this disease. That's because the female vaginal, urinary, and anal openings are close together. Any bacteria from the anal area can easily be swept up into the urethra and make their way to the bladder.

Symptoms of bladder infection include:

- urinating many times throughout the day
- intense desire to urinate even when there's nothing to come out
- cloudy urine
- burning sensation while urinating
- possible abdominal pain
- possible blood in the urine

If you think you have a bladder infection, see a doctor immediately. She or he will take a urine sample and have it cultured in a lab to confirm that you really do have a bladder infection. If you do have an infection, you'll be given an antibiotic. If the pain is intense, your doctor may also prescribe a pain reliever. Usually, the pain clears up within 24 hours. However, it's essential that you take the full dosage of medicine given to you by the doctor. If you abandon the medication before you've taken the full amount, you're putting yourself at risk for another bout of infection!

Ovarian Cysts

Ovarian cysts are benign (noncancerous) growths in the ovaries. Almost 50 percent of all tumors found in the ovaries are benign cysts.

What is a cyst anyway? It's a self-contained sac that contains fluid and sometimes solid matter. It can be very small, or it can grow to be as large as or bigger than an orange.

An ovarian cyst can result when the ovary fails to release the egg during ovulation. The stimulated follicle swells and gets filled with fluid to form a cyst.

How can you tell if you have a cyst? Often doctors find

them during routine exams. They may be able to feel the cyst by pressing on your lower abdomen.

You may also suffer from certain symptoms, particularly recurring or chronic abdominal pain or menstrual irregularities.

Ovarian cysts are usually nothing to worry about. Often they break open and disappear on their own. Sometimes, however, doctors will remove a cyst or try and shrink it with birth control hormones. If you have a cyst, your doctor will know the best way to take care of it.

Breast Lumps

Sometimes just reading the words *breast lump* can make you panic because you know that a lump can mean cancer. Don't worry. Breast cancer in girls your age is very rare. In fact, *less than one percent* of breast lumps in adolescents are cancerous.

If you do feel a lump, what could it mean? Some girls' breasts get lumpy before their periods due to hormones. Some girls may have exceptionally lumpy breasts to begin with, a condition known as fibrocystic disease. The lump you feel may also just be a natural part of your breast. For example, milk ducts, the breastbone, ribs, and underlying muscle can all feel like lumps.

With time, as you get more used to the feel of your breasts, you'll be able to tell the difference between normal lumps and any new lumps. In the meantime, however, if you discover a lump that stays for several weeks, see a doctor just to be safe and to reassure yourself.

Your Family History

Some families are more prone to develop cancer than others. If you belong to a family in which one or more members have had cancer (especially close relatives), pay special attention to any lumps.

WHAT IS CANCER?

Cancer is a disease in which the body's cells become abnormal and begin to grow uncontrollably. Normally, the cells that make up the body reproduce themselves in a very orderly manner. However, sometimes cells will grow into a mass of tissue called a tumor. Some tumors are benign; others are cancerous.

Benign tumors may require surgical removal, but they do not invade other tissues of the body and usually are relatively harmless. However, cancerous tumors (called malignant tumors) invade and destroy normal tissue. The cancerous cells break away from the malignant tumor and spread through the blood and lymphatic systems of the body to other areas. This process is called *metastasis*. Sometimes cancer grows and spreads rapidly; other times it takes years.

Breast cancer can spread from the breast to the lymph nodes in the armpit, neck, and chest, and eventually to other parts of the body via the bloodstream.

Scoliosis

This is a condition in which the spine curves to the side instead of growing straight. It usually becomes apparent in young people between the ages of 10 and 16, and it affects girls more than boys.

Scoliosis isn't something you can "catch." You're either born with the tendency to develop it or not. It shows up during puberty because the growth spurt makes the condition more apparent.

Often scoliosis is discovered by routine school screenings,

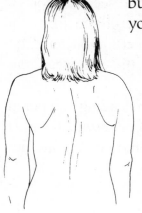

but it must be evaluated by a doctor. If you're found to have scoliosis, don't panic. Of all the kids identified as having scoliosis, only a few will require treatment.

Those who do need treatment can often have their condition corrected, either through wearing a back brace or, in severe cases, through surgery. (During surgery, an adjustable rod is implanted in the back to help straighten the spine.)

Strep Throat

It starts with a sore throat, then grows into full-grown misery. Strep throat can really lay you low. Peak months to catch the disease are November through May. And, as luck would have it, if you're between the ages of 5 and 15, you're at the biggest risk for strep throat!

Sometimes it's hard to tell if you have just a cold or the real thing. Besides a sore throat, strep throat can also bring on these symptoms:

- fever
- pus on the tonsils
- redness on the back of your throat
- stomachaches
- nausea and vomiting
- a red skin rash

A runny nose and a cough are usually not part of the strep infection. Sometimes the only symptoms a person suffering from strep throat will feel is a fever and a sore throat.

If you think you might have strep throat, see a doctor. He or she will take a sampling (a throat culture) from the inflamed area and run a test on it to detect the bacteria that cause strep. If you do have strep throat, the doctor will prescribe an antibiotic to get you well.

Left untreated, strep throat can worsen, leading to a potentially dangerous complication called *rheumatic fever*. Rheumatic fever can affect the joints, heart, kidneys, and nervous system.

Mononucleosis

Mononucleosis (mono) is often called the kissing disease. But you really don't have to kiss someone to catch it. That's an old wives' tale. In fact, you can have very close contact with a person who has mono and *not* catch it.

Doctors know mono is caused by a virus, but they're not really sure how people catch it. Some research suggests that people who are tired or run-down are at greater risk for mono.

What are the typical symptoms in a young person?

The main one is exhaustion. A person with mono often craves and needs a lot of sleep. Other symptoms may include:

- swollen lymph glands in the neck

- headaches

- sore throat

- in some cases, a skin rash

- enlarged liver and/or spleen

Sometimes it's hard to tell if you really have mono or you're just run-down. If you suspect you might have mono, see a doctor.

Once you're at the doctor's office, he or she will give you a blood test to determine if you have the disease. If you have mono, there's not much you can do but get a lot of rest and eat well. Recovery time varies from person to person. Sometimes mono will keep you sidelined for only a week or two. Other times it can take months to get over it.

Pierced Ear Infections

You sure looked great when you first got your ears pierced. You couldn't wait to show off your pair of gold studs! But now, two months down the road, your earlobes are scratchy and red, and the holes filled with pus or a sticky, crusty liquid.

What's going on? It sounds like your ear holes are infected.

What causes an infection? Often, it's a result of not taking good enough care of your ears.

When you have your ears pierced, your ears are punctured. Like any wound, these small puncture holes are subject to infection. If you don't keep the area clean enough, especially when the holes are healing, they can become infected. Some materials in the earrings can also irritate your skin.

To avoid any infection:

- Keep your earlobes and earrings clean. Dip a cotton ball in some peroxide and dab the front and back of your ear-lobe every morning before putting your earrings in and at night after you've taken them out.

- If your ears are newly pierced, twist the earrings every day to keep the air circulating under the earrings. This also makes sure that the earrings aren't pressing too tightly into your ear.

- If your skin around the hole starts to get red and irritated, remove your earrings immediately. If you keep them in, the infection may grow worse. The skin may become so soft and swollen with irritation that the earring sinks into your skin, and eventually a doctor has to dig it out.

- Stick with earrings made of material you know you're not sensitive to.

- Take out your earrings each night.

- Avoid wearing heavy earrings, as these can really put a strain on your ear holes.

See a doctor if you're doing all you can to keep your ear holes clean, but they're still getting infected.

Sunburn

You didn't mean to roast your face for six hours in the sun, but playing volleyball at the lake was so much fun, you forgot to put on a hat or sunscreen.

Now you're paying the price. Your face is so red it looks like a ripe tomato. It hurts to smile, let alone laugh.

To avoid getting overdone in the sun, apply a sunscreen 30 minutes before going outside. Make sure whatever product you choose has a sun protection factor (SPF) of at least 15. An SPF level measures the amount of time you can stay in the sun without getting burned. For example, an SPF of 15 means you can stay in the sun 15 times longer than you normally could and not get a sunburn. If you're particularly fair, be sure to reapply the sunscreen every hour or so. Of course, if the sunscreen has washed off, be sure to reapply it.

Also, choose a sunscreen with both ultraviolet A (UVA) and ultraviolet B (UVB) protection. Many screens protect you from just the UVB (the "burning rays"). However, the UVA rays penetrate even deeper and can do more damage to your skin, increasing the risk of skin cancer and wrinkling.

In addition, avoid the sun when the sun's rays are at their most direct—from 11 A.M. to 3 P.M. each day. And cover up with a hat for extra protection.

Avoid tanning salons altogether.

Depression

Why are we including depression with the above medical problems? While depression affects how you feel, it can also affect your body. It can exhaust you and cause headaches, stomachaches, and other physical symptoms.

Depression is a feeling of deep sadness and despair. People who are depressed may feel as if there's nothing to look forward to or live for.

Depression affects millions of people each year. It can strike old people, middle-aged people, and young people like you. You may be prone to it especially during puberty, when you're going through so many confusing changes.

It's natural to feel depressed when you go through a tragedy, like if your parents are divorcing, or a loss, like when your best friend moves across the country.

But if you feel depressed for no reason, or if your depression lasts for weeks and months, you need help.

We don't want to scare you, but sometimes kids get so depressed that they consider or even attempt suicide. Teens, in fact, have a very high suicide rate.

How do you know if you (or a friend) are depressed? If you answer yes to most of these questions, you may be depressed:

- Do you feel tired a lot, no matter how much sleep you get?

- Do you find that it's hard to get up enough energy to do the simplest task, such as feeding your cat or talking to a friend?

- Do you find yourself wanting to be alone more, instead of being with your friends or family?

- Have you lost interest in all the things you used to love, like playing tennis or going out for ice cream with your big sister or even listening to your favorite CD?

- Do you find yourself wishing you could be someone else?

- Have you quit caring about how you look or stopped eating healthfully?

- Are you crying a lot, usually for no reason?

- Have you either lost or gained a lot of weight recently?

- Do you feel hopeless and helpless, as if there's nothing to look forward to and nothing you can do to change anything anyway?

If you did answer yes to several of these questions, first find a trusted friend or adult with whom you can share your feelings. See if that helps how you feel.

The next step is tougher, but you can do it. Through school or your parents, find a counselor you can talk to. Sharing your thoughts with a counselor can really help you figure out your feelings and make you feel better.

Depression is too big a problem to handle on your own. Don't be afraid to seek some advice and comfort.

Your First Visit to the Gynecologist

Now that you're getting older, your parents or family doctor may suggest you have a gynecological examination. Gynecology is a branch of medicine specializing in the female reproductive system. In a gynecological exam, the doctor looks at your reproductive organs, both internal and external. While that may sound confusing or even scary, seeing a *gynecologist* is a good first step to insuring your health as you grow into womanhood. Many gynecologists also practice "obstetrics"—which means they monitor the health of pregnant women and then deliver their babies. These dual-specialty doctors are frequently referred to by the letters: OB/GYN, which stands for Obstetrics/Gynecology. Some gynecologists specialize in treating young women like you and are called "pediatric gynecologists." Your gynecologist will likely be the same doctor who treats your mother or a physician with whom your family doctor or health insurance company is quite familiar. Although it can seem embarrassing to have your private parts examined, remember that your doctor is a professional who is accustomed to this type of work. He or she is not judging how your body looks, just whether or not it is healthy. However, if you feel highly uncomfortable with your gynecologist, or if you wonder whether his or her behavior is appropriate, be sure to talk about it with a parent, family doctor, or school nurse! An initial gynecological examination may take an hour or longer, because so many important steps are involved. Here is a step-by-step guide of what you can expect during your first exam:

1. Before the Visit

Your first exam will be quicker and more efficient with a little preparation on your part. Be prepared with the following information that your doctor will need to know:

- your medical information, including any histories of serious illnesses and surgeries
- the history of your periods (when you began having a period, the average length, and the date of your last period)
- your family's medical history (your mom or dad can help you put this information together)

- questions you have about your body or changes you are experiencing, both physical and emotional

Of course, you'll want to shower and wear clean under-clothing to your examination. If you are on or start your period on your appointment date, call your doctor's office and alert them. Your gynecologist may choose to reschedule your appointment to a time when you are off your period.

2. THE PRE-EXAMINATION

In the waiting room, you'll sign in and fill out paperwork about your personal and medical information. A nurse or medical assistant will then call your name and escort you from the waiting room. Your mother may accompany you, but many doctors don't allow friends or male relatives into examining rooms.

The nurse will have you step on a weight scale and check your height. She may then ask you to "void" (urinate) into a specimen cup. You may worry about this step, since it can be messy or embarrassing. Just follow the nurse's instructions and remember that it's a routine procedure for the office personnel. A blood sample may also be drawn at this time.

Next, the nurse will escort you into a private examining room, and have you disrobe and wear a paper or cotton examining gown. When the nurse returns, she will take your "vitals." This means your blood pressure, pulse, and body temperature will be checked and recorded on your medical chart. The nurse will ask if you are allergic to any medications, and note your answer on the chart, as well.

3. THE CLINICAL INTERVIEW

The first time you meet with your gynecologist, he or she will take a medical history of you and your family. This clinical interview is an excellent opportunity for you to discuss any questions or concerns you may have about your anatomy.

Your doctor will also ask about your sexual history to insure you receive appropriate medical care. If you've ever had sexual intercourse or think it's a possibility in the near future, be completely honest with your doctor. Share any fears you may have about confidentiality, so that you and your doctor can discuss the extent to which your parents will be involved in your medical care. If you are sexually active, your doctor will discuss birth control and sexually transmitted diseases with you. It's important to pay close attention and to follow any advice given by your doctor.

Your doctor will probably ask about any menstrual problems or discomfort you may have experienced. If you've had any menstrual or urinary-tract related pain or concerns, this is a good time to discuss them.

Finally, your doctor will likely spend some time chatting with you to find out more about your personal life. Your doctor isn't being a snoop; he or she wants to know about you and your lifestyle habits for a couple of reasons.

First, your gynecologist realizes how stress, diet, and nutrition affect health and menstrual cycles. So, your doctor needs to know about such factors in your life.

Second, you'll likely be a long-term patient of your gynecologist. This doctor will see you through adolescence and into adulthood. He or she may even deliver any babies you have in the future! In addition, many women go to their gynecologist for routine medical issues unrelated to reproductive health. No wonder, then, that it's so important for the two of you to talk and feel comfortable with one another!

After the clinical interview, your doctor may leave you alone in the examining room for a few moments before the actual gynecological examination. A nurse may ask if you can urinate again, as an empty bladder makes the examination more efficient.

4. THE EXAM

Your doctor or nurse will ask you to lie down on the examining table. To let go of any anxiety of embarrassment, take a deep breath, focus your eyes on an object in the room, or hold the nurse's hand. The more relaxed you are, the more comfortable and thorough your examination will be.

Your doctor will likely begin by checking each breast for abnormal lumps. Don't worry that your doctor can feel your rapidly beating heart; he or she is a professional who routinely conducts breast examinations.

Next, they will ask you to put your feet into stirrups and relax so that your legs spread apart. They will drape a sheet across your legs. The doctor then shines a bright light to conduct the pelvic examination, which consists of four steps.

First, the doctor inspects your vulva, or external genitalia, for signs of normal or abnormal development.

Next, the doctor inserts a plastic or metal device called a speculum into your vaginal opening. This allows your doctor to check your cervix and vaginal walls. Alert your doctor to any painful sensations, as pain can signal the presence of inflammation or other medical conditions warranting treatment.

After inserting the speculum, your doctor will conduct a Pap test (named for its inventor Dr. Papanicolaou). In a Pap test, your gynecologist gently scrapes a layer of your cervix cells and transfers them to a glass slide for microscopic examination to make sure all cells are normal and healthy.

Then the doctor will examine your uterus, fallopian tubes, and ovaries. The gynecologist will insert two gloved fingers into the vagina while pressing down with the other hand. This procedure may feel uncomfortable, and your doctor will ask you to speak up if you experience any pain. Try to relax your abdomen as much as possible, both to reduce discomfort and to help your doctor accurately examine your ovaries.

The final step is a rectal exam. Your doctor will insert one gloved finger into the rectum opening and one into the vagina. As with the other steps, you may feel pressure, discomfort, or embarrassment, but deep breathing will help you relax. Plus, keep in mind that your examination is almost over!

FOLLOW-UP CARE

You won't see your gynecologist for a while, unless your tests suggest a problem, you get ill, or become sexually active. Most doctors recommend having a gynecological examination every three years until the age of 40. Between these visits, it's important to give yourself a monthly breast exam. Once you become sexually active, you'll also need an annual Pap exam. You'll also have to check in with the gynecologist once a year if you choose a medical prescription for birth control.

Hey, Tomorrow!

"What will I be? A nurse, an animal doctor? No, besides that, who will I be, what sort of woman?"
She startled herself. "Me, a woman?"

—Katie John in Mary Calhoun's *Honestly Katie John!*

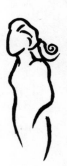

When you're just sitting there—alone in your room or in the middle of class—do you ever suddenly get a shiver of excitement about the future?

Maybe you've just gotten a mental glimpse of yourself in 5, 10, or 15 years. There you are, walking through the bustling city of Paris on the way to an important international business meeting.

Or maybe you see yourself entering an old, ivy-covered college building, books in hand and surrounded by friends.

Or perhaps you see yourself in a cozy house complete with a white picket fence, a child in your arms, and a handsome husband cooking dinner in the kitchen.

Whatever you see when you look into the future, it's within your grasp. In the years ahead, you'll have opportunities for love, travel, education, career, and happy times spent with good friends and family. You can do whatever you want to do, and be who you want to be.

In the meantime, it won't always be easy growing up. But it does get easier as you get the hang of it.

It's true that once you enter puberty, things will never be the same again in your life. But you know what? You really wouldn't want them to be!

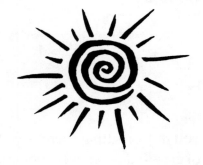

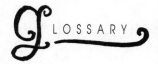

GLOSSARY

aerobic (ihr-OH-bihk): Any activity that increases breathing and heart paces to a target heart rate. Aerobic exercises efficiently burn body fat.

alveoli (al-vee-OH-ly): The tiny structures in the breast that produce milk for babies.

amenorrhea (uh-men-uh-REE-uh): Absence of the regular monthly menstrual cycle.

androgens (AN-druh-jenz): Male sex hormones that both men and women produce. During puberty, they are the hormones that turn on the sweat glands among other changes.

anorexia nervosa (an-uh-REK-see-uh ner-VOHS-uh): An eating disorder that causes people to starve themselves in order to stay thin.

areola (uh-ree-OH-luh): The round, pinkish-brown area around the nipple on a breast.

breast (BREST): One of two organs located on the chest wall containing the glands that produce milk for newborns. Girls begin developing breasts during puberty.

bulimia (buh-LEEM-ee-uh): An eating disorder that causes people to binge on food, then purge it, which usually involves vomiting and excess use of laxatives.

cellulite (SELL-you-lite): A non-medical term for ordinary body fat distributed in ways that appear as dimples. Female hormones sometimes create the appearance of cellulite on the back of thighs and buttocks.

cervix (SER-viks): The low end of the uterus that joins to the vagina.

clitoris (KLIT-uh-rus): A small, knoblike structure in the female's vulva.

corpus luteum (KOR-pus LOOT-ee-um): A yellowish tissue from which the hormone progesterone is released after ovulation.

ductus deferens (DUK-tuhs DEF-uh-renz): A tube that carries sperm from the epididymis to the ejaculatory duct.

dysmenorrhea (diss-men-uh-REE-uh): Painful periods.

ejaculation (ih-jak-yuh-LAY-shun): The sudden discharge of semen out of the end of a male's penis when he reaches sexual climax.

endometrium (en-doh-MEE-tree-um): The innermost lining of the uterus. During the menstrual cycle, tissue builds up on this lining. If an egg isn't fertilized, the tissue is shed during menstruation. During pregnancy, the endometrium helps to nourish the baby.

epididymis (ep-uh-DID-uh-mas): The mass of tubes that carries sperm from the testes to the ductus deferens.

erection (ih-REK-shun): The swelling and hardening of the penis when a male becomes sexually excited. The swelling is caused by blood flowing into the tissues of the penis.

estrogen (ESS-truh-jen): One of several hormones that causes many of the physical changes girls experience during puberty. Estrogen is produced by the ovaries.

fallopian tube (fuh-LOH-pee-un TOOB): One of two tubes

leading from the top of the uterus, whose opened end is positioned right next to one of the two ovaries. When an egg is released from an ovary, it is swept into a fallopian tube and then into the uterus. The fallopian tube is usually where an egg is fertilized by a sperm.

fertilization (fert-ul-u-ZAY-shun): The process in which a male sperm joins with a female egg. Pregnancy begins at fertilization.

fimbria (FIM-bree-uh): The bordering fringe around the entrance of the fallopian tubes.

follicle (FAHL-uh-kul): One of many structural units within the ovaries that holds and protects a developing egg cell, as well as produces estrogen.

genitalia (jen-uh-TAYL-yuh): The sexual and reproductive organs. In males, the genitalia include the penis, scrotum, and testicles. In females, they include the vagina, uterus, and ovaries.

gynecologist (gi-neh-KAH-lah-gist): A medical doctor specializing in the health and treatment of women's reproductive systems. Also called an OB/GYN, when the doctor dual-specializes in obstetrics (the care of pregnant women and baby delivery).

hormones (HOR-mohnz): A wide variety of protein molecules that are produced and released from special glands in your body.

hymen (HY-mun): The membranous tissue that partially covers the vaginal opening.

hypothalamus (hy-poh-THAL-uh-mus): A structure in the brain that produces the substance Gonadotropin releasing hormone (GnRh), which is involved in initiating puberty.

iron-deficiency anemia (I-ern DEE-fish-en-see uh-NEE-mee-uh): A disease of decreased red blood cell mass caused by lack of iron in the body.

labia majora (LAY-bee-uh muh-JOR-uh): The outer lips of the vulva, outside the vagina.

labia minora (LAY-bee-uh muh-NOR-uh): The lips inside the outer lips that are on either side of the vaginal opening.

lobes (LOHBZ): Several separate milk-producing units that are found in each breast.

menarche (MEN-ar-kee): The onset of menstruation.

menstrual cycle (MEN-strool SY-kul): The monthly female reproductive cycle.

milk ducts: (MILK DUKTS): The milk-carrying tubes that lead from the alveoli or milk glands to small openings on the surface of the nipples.

myometrium (my-oh-MEE-tree-um): The muscular middle layer of the uterine wall, which contracts during menstruation. During delivery of a baby, the contractions of this muscle help to push out the baby.

obesity (O-BEES-ih-tee): Excessive body weight caused by overeating, heredity, a nonactive lifestyle, or a combination of any of the above. Obesity can harm a person both physically and psychologically.

osteoporosis (AHSS-tee-oh-puh-ROH-sus): A loss of bone volume, usually seen in older women, which results in brittle bones.

ovary (OHV-uh-ree): One of two almond-shaped organs in the female reproductive system. The two ovaries contain all the egg cells needed for reproduction for a lifetime.

ovulation (AHV-yoo-lay-shun): The process in which an egg is released from one of the ovaries and begins to travel to the uterus. Ovulation usually occurs once a month.

ovum (OH-vum): A female's reproductive cell, or egg.

pectoral (PEK-tuh-rel): Referring to the chest area.

penis (PEE-nus): A male's external sexual organ.

pituitary gland (pih-TOO-e-ter-ee GLAND): The structure within the brain that produces several hormones, including FSH and LH.

progesterone (proh-JES-tuh-rohn): A hormone produced by the corpus luteum, progesterone causes some of the physical changes you experience during puberty. It's also important in regulating a girl's monthly menstrual cycle and in maintaining pregnancy.

prostaglandins (prahss-tuh-GLAN-dunz): Hormonelike chemicals that cause the muscle in the uterus to contract during menstruation.

prostate gland (PRAHSS-tayt GLAND): The gland that surrounds the male urethra just below the urinary bladder. The prostate gland secretes liquid into the seminal fluid during ejaculation.

puberty (PYOO-bert-ee): The physical and emotional changes that take place in everybody between childhood and adulthood.

scrotum (SKROH-tum): The sack of skin that hangs down behind a male's penis and holds the testicles.

semen (SEE-mun): A liquid made up of sperm and fluids. When a male has an ejaculation, semen comes out of the tip of the penis.

serosa (suh-ROH-zuh): The smooth outer covering of the uterus.

serotonin (sihr-uh-TO-nihn): A brain chemical responsible for regulating mood and energy levels. Lifestyle habits, including diet, exercise, stress, and sleep affect serotonin.

speculum (SPE-kyou-luhm): A plastic or metal device used by gynecologists during a pelvic examination. The doctor inserts the speculum into the vaginal opening to conduct an examination and collect cell specimens.

sperm (SPERM): A male's reproductive cell, also called spermatozoon.

staphylococcus aureus (staf-uh-loh-KAHK-us OR-ee-us): The bacterium that probably causes toxic shock syndrome. It lives on the skin and in the body's warm, moist cavities.

STD: An acronym for sexually transmitted diseases, an STD is a disease that is passed from person to person usually by sexual intercourse or other intimate contact. Some STDs include genital warts, syphilis, and AIDS.

target heart rate: This is the rate at which your heart should beat during exercise. To find your THR, subtract your age from 220. Then, multiply it by .75. This will be your THR.

testicles (TESS-tih-kulz): In a male, the two small egg-shaped organs inside the scrotum that produce sperm.

toxic shock syndrome (TOKS-ic SHOK SIN-druhm): Also known as TSS, toxic shock syndrome is a disease that has been linked to tampon use. (However, TSS has occurred in men, as well as in women not menstruating.)

urethra (yoo-REE-thruh): The tube leading from the bladder to the outside of the body through which urine passes.

uterus (YOOT-e-rus): An upside-down pear shape structure located in the pelvis, this organ is where a baby grows.

vagina (vah-JY-nah): Another female sexual organ, the vagina is the canal that leads from the uterus to the outside of the body. During menstruation, blood and tissue pass through the vagina.

vaginitis (va-ji-NY-tiss): An inflammation of the vagina, common in females.

vulva (VUL-vah): The genital organs on the outside of the female body.

zygote (ZY-goht): A fertilized egg.

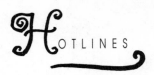

Hotlines

If you or someone you know is in trouble, don't try to deal with it alone. Free, confidential help is just a phone call away. Most of these hotlines have toll-free numbers, so there's no reason not to reach out if you know you need help. Here are some hotlines staffed by trained counselors who can provide comfort, referrals to local professionals, and information.

Note: In cases of immediate physical trauma, danger, or suicidal behavior, dial 911 or 0 for assistance right away.

Suicide Prevention Hotlines

National Runaway and Suicide Hotline
1-800-621-4000
Provides 24-hour crisis intervention and referrals.

Kid Save
1-800-543-7283
Provides 24-hour crisis intervention and referrals for all mental health issues related to children and young adults.

Substance Abuse Hotline

National Institute of Drug Abuse
Parklawn Building
5600 Fishers Lane, Room 10A-39
Rockville, MD 20852
1-800-662-4357
Provides 24-hour crisis counseling, referrals, and information related to alcoholism or substance abuse.

Covenant House Hotline
1-800-999-9999
Provides 24-hour crisis intervention and referrals, especially for young people who have or who are considering, running away from home.

Sexual Assault Hotlines

Rape, Abuse, and Incest National Network (RAIN)
252 10th St. NE
Washington, DC 20002
1-800-656-4673 (HOPE)
This 24-hour hotline automatically connects you to a counselor in an area near to you.

Child Help, USA
6463 Independence Ave.
Woodland Hills, CA 91367
1-800-422-4453 (1-800-4-A-CHILD)
A 24-hour hotline, referral, and information center specializing in child abuse and sexual crimes against children.

Sexual Assault Victims Hotline
1520 Eighth Ave.
Meridan, MI 39302
1-800-643-6250
This 24-hour hotline provides counseling and local referrals.

REFERRAL AGENCIES

The purpose of these agencies is to refer you to a local group or counselor who can help you. Usually, these agencies are not equipped to give crisis counseling over the telephone. Many of these referral centers provide mental health information, pamphlets, or reports that can be mailed to you free of charge.

Child Abuse and Domestic Violence Referral Agencies

National Organization for Victims Assistance (NOVA)
1757 Park Road NW
Washington, DC 20010
1-800-879-6682 (1-800-TRY-NOVA)
Provides 24-hour referrals, and victims rights information for anyone who is a victim of a crime, including child abuse, domestic violence, and sexual assault.

National Victims Center
2111 Wilson Blvd., Suite 300
Arlington, VA 22201
1-800-394-2255 (1-800-FYI-CALL)
Provides referrals to local domestic violence shelters, open 9 to 5 Eastern Standard Time.

Eating Disorders Referral Agencies

Renfrew Eating Disorder Center
1-800-RENFREW
Provides 24-hour referrals to local eating disorder treatment centers.

The American Anorexia/Bulimia Association
(212) 501-8351
Provides referrals to local eating disorder therapists, as well as information.

The National Association of Anorexia Nervosa and Associated Disorders
(847) 831-3438
Provides referrals to local eating disorder therapists, as well as information.

Mental Health Referral Agencies
National Alliance for the Mentally Ill
2101 Wilson Blvd., Suite 302
Arlington, VA 22201
1-800-950-6264
Makes referrals to local support groups and counselors.

National Foundation for Depressive Illness
P.O. Box 2257
New York, NY 10116
1-800-248-4344
Makes referrals to local organizations and counselors specializing in treating depression.

National Mental Health Association
1021 Prince St.
Alexandria, VA 22314
1-800-969-6642
Makes referrals to local support groups and counselors.

Substance Abuse Referral Agencies

Alcoholics Anonymous
General Service Office
475 Riverside Drive
New York, NY 10115
Call directory assistance for the Alcoholic's Anonymous nearest you, or call (212) 870-3400 for referrals and information related to alcoholism.

Cocaine Abuse Referral Agencies

Cocaine Anonymous
1-800-347-8998
Provides 24-hour referrals and information related to cocaine abuse and addiction.

National Cocaine Abuse Hotline
1-800-COCAINE
Provides 24-hour referrals and information related to cocaine abuse and addiction.

Medical Help and Information Referrals
American Diabetes Association Diabetes Information Service Center
1660 Duke St., Alexandria, VA 22314
1-800-232-3472

$\mathcal{I}$ NDEX

ABOUT THE AUTHORS

The author of the preteen advice book, *Ask Allie*, **Alison Bell** is a former advice columnist and associate managing editor at *'TEEN* magazine. Her other midgrade titles include *The Dream Scene* and *How to Analyze Handwriting*. She has written for such other national magazines as *YM, Women's Sports and Fitness,* and *New Body*. She lives with her husband and two children in Venice, California.

A graduate of New York University School of Medicine, **Lisa Rooney, M.D.,** is a pediatrician practicing in Stamford, Connecticut, as well as a fellow of the American Academy of Pediatrics. In her private practice, Dr. Rooney especially enjoys counseling adolescents on their health care needs. She lives in Greenwich, Connecticut, with her husband and three children.